THE
PARADOX
OF
HEALING

*Transforming your relationship
with illness*

MICHAEL GREENWOOD
and
PETER NUNN

PRION

Fourth edition (revised) 1996

First published in Great Britain 1996 by PRION
32–34 Gordon House Road,
London NW5 1LP

First published in 1994 Canada by Paradox Publishers

A catalogue record of this book can be obtained
from the British Library

ISBN 1-85375-216-9

Cover design by Design Revolution
Printed and bound in Great Britain by
Biddles Ltd., Guildford & Kings Lynn

CONTENTS

Index

INTRODUCTION

Medicine is not the solution to illness, it is the illness

The Paradox of Healing takes a look at the problem of chronic illness and chronic pain and offers new insight into their origins, their meaning in our lives and the very real opportunity they present for our profound and far-reaching healing.

Chronic conditions are by definition those which do not respond to our treatment of them. And because we cannot cure them, these intractable problems can offer an opportunity to both doctors and patients to re-examine the whole approach to sickness, pain and disease commonly taken by our society.

Trained as physicians, Peter Nunn and I were rigorously schooled in the beliefs which underlie conventional medicine and its techniques. Naturally, when we started out, it was far from our minds ever to question those beliefs, backed up as they were by the weight of scientific authority, vast pharmacies of drugs, armies of specialists and researchers, and increasingly sophisticated equipment and techniques.

What we have learned through the years, however, is that chronic pain or illness are catch-22 situations. Faced with the uncomfortable truth that there seemed to be no adequate explanation or treatment for their pain, we watched many patients confront the fact that medicine cannot cure many illnesses which are not "rational," because scientific medicine can only deal with the rational.

What the chronically ill really face, we discovered, is the problem of paradox. The Oxford Dictionary defines paradox as a "self-contradictory, essentially absurd statement; a person or thing conflicting with preconceived notions of what is reasonable or possible."

All of us sooner or later face a situation which defies a rational solution, a totally unsolvable problem which leaves us no option but to come to terms with the fact that we *just don't know*. If we are always sick or in pain, we are sooner or later challenged to accept the unacceptable—to reconcile ourselves with the great mystery of our existence. No wonder many of us, rather than grapple seriously with the problem, look for an easy way out!

The simplest way to avoid paradox is to deny its existence by denying half of its self-contradictory proposition. We may be chronically ill, but someone somewhere must have a cure. Denial is the easiest and most attractive response. It allows us to continue to think that we have rational control of our lives, and avoid the real issue posed by the contradiction we face—the unpleasant thought that there may be nobody who can cure us, and no way to get rid of our illness, that it is in fact a real part of us, however unlikeable.

At the root of our modern Western society and of our medicine, unfortunately, is exactly this sort of collective denial. But such denial carries severe penalties. Denying half of reality results in the sacrifice of half of who we are. Further, since the rejected half is hidden by a wall of denial, few of us ever realize our loss, and so condemn ourselves to living limited lives, with no awareness of our larger potential. We are, of course, only fooling ourselves. Such limited solutions cannot last. Sooner or later, life corrects the imbalance.

In the meantime, putting off the confrontation with paradox worsens our situation. As the denial grows, we get sicker, and if the paradox is continually denied, it will keep growing. Eventually, we are confronted by contradictions so huge we may die. It is at this point that we have an opportunity to regain our wholeness and our health.

Conventional medicine, however, cannot help us. It is caught in the same trap of denial as we are. As a society, we have long since convinced ourselves that reason is superior to emotion because feelings fail to obey the dictates of logic, and are thus irrational. This circular argument permits the rational to create the world in its own image— the very essence of denial. The result is that the notion that the irrational could affect the disease process is thoroughly discouraged in modern medicine as "unscientific." Illnesses which have their roots in the irrational must therefore be dismissed as unreal.

As practising physicians, however, we have come to believe that the denial of feelings—the irrational part of ourselves—will eventually *lead to* illness, or chronic pain. And, further, we have seen how far grappling with our despair and our personal paradoxes can lead to healing.

In fact, we now believe that hidden in the physical manifestation of much of the pain and illness which present themselves to the physician lies an awesome truth. Our experience has led us to conclude that a profound change is required in our society's approach to medicine, one that embraces our whole being, and emphasizes transformation over treatment. This, we believe, is the medicine of the future.

By ignoring the emotions, conventional medicine wastes time, money and energy trying to find rational explanations for disease when there may be none to find. And the enormous effort sometimes undertaken to make a diagnosis may itself, paradoxically, promote illness.

Consider a young man in stressful circumstances who comes into the physician's office complaining of chest pain. The young man is worried that the pain might be due to a "bad heart." Any thorough physician would be expected to initiate a series of tests—an ECG, blood tests, chest X-ray and an exercise stress test, perhaps—to rule out coronary disease. Such tests are bound to increase the young man's anxiety. If the results are "equivocal," as they so often are, the chances are that he will be referred to a heart specialist, who has little choice under the circumstances but to suggest coronary angiography.

The actual situation is that of a young man who is afraid that he is sick. He does not have heart disease, he has fear, which may have been initiated by other circumstances in his life. He has focussed this fear on his heart, and his doctor reinforces it by initiating tests for heart disease.

In truth, the doctor also has fear—fear that he or she might miss a diagnosis and become vulnerable to a lawsuit. This apprehension may dissuade a doctor from taking a commonsense approach to help the young man deal with his anxiety. Thus a lot of tests which are purportedly performed to alleviate anxiety in the patient in fact only relieve anxiety in the physician. In any case, neither the doctor nor the specialist has the time or training to help the patient deal with the root of his anxiety, since fear is not considered a physical illness and is therefore not "real."

Modern medicine has neither the capacity to deal with anxiety and fear, nor with the mind–body connection which they imply. When confronted with anxiety in their offices, many physicians resort to drugs to suppress its symptoms, rather than try to discover its meaning. It is a rare physician indeed who searches beyond the symptoms of physical illnesses to find the impact of ideas and feelings on a patient's physical health.

One solution to this situation is to educate doctors and patients to adopt a holistic approach—one that takes the whole patient, and not simply the ailment, into account. Holism can answer paradox because it accepts both the rational and irrational in us. It allows sufferers of chronic stress-related illness to come to grips with the problems posed by their lives and painfully reflected in their bodies and to embark on a process of personal transformation that will lead them ultimately to heal themselves.

This transformation is not simply a change of habits. Transformation is a profound change of heart made possible by the renewed sense of being which comes from facing the paradoxical nature of our existence. Nor is transformation a new idea. It is part of our cultural heritage—the motivating force at the centre of many of the ancient myths which shaped our early literature and continue to influence our understanding of our lives, and is more familiar still in the fairy tales that fascinated us as children. Its application to medicine, however, for those of us used to an emphasis on scientific, rational approaches to illness, is not easy to grasp.

In fact, mythology is an excellent approach to healing. Myths relate the rational to the irrational, and individuals to their cultures, connecting the personal to the supra-personal without moralizing or teaching any particular doctrine. In other words, they simply and complexly describe the greater universe in which we are all embedded; and in them we may learn to recognize the "other," the dark side of ourselves, and encounter life through our hearts rather than through our intellects.

Read as guides to ourselves, many of these familiar stories capture the magic of the transformational journey which is central to the healing experience, and can open up a whole new understanding of the meaning of illness and health, and help us start our own journey.

The Paradox of Healing is both a challenge to conventional medicine and an inspiration to transform ourselves, medicine and society. ——*M.G.*

Chapter One

A KING AND HIS THREE SONS

The choice to die is the choice to live

There once was a king who had three sons. As each reached his majority, the king asked him to go out into the world to prove himself. In this way, the old king hoped to discover which of the princes would be most worthy to succeed him.

The first son rode out on his horse, and after a time he came to a signpost which pointed three ways. To the left, it read: "If you go this way, there will be enough food for your horse, but not enough for you." To the right, the sign informed the traveller: "If you go this way, there will be enough food for you, but your horse will go hungry." The third sign, which pointed straight ahead, said bluntly: "If you go this way you will die."

The first son chose the road to the right, rationalizing that if he were well fed he would be able to handle any problems which might crop up. In any case, if anyone were going to starve it was not going to be he. He rode on until his horse could go no further, and leaving it at the side of the road, continued on foot.

Eventually, high in the mountains, the prince came across a copper snake which, because he had found little else, he decided to take home to his father. Unfortunately, the king was enraged at a gift of so little value—in his opinion, snakes were nothing but trouble. And so the first son was imprisoned for lack of achievement.

Soon after this, the second son reached the age of majority and was sent out into the world. He likewise came to to the signpost. Being of quite a different disposition than his older brother, he chose the left fork, rationalizing that his horse's strength was more important than his own on such a journey, and that in any case, if the worse came to the worst, he could always eat grass, or even the horse itself.

After a few hours, he came to a village where there lived a beautiful maiden. This maiden stopped the handsome stranger as he rode by her house, and invited him in, promising him all kinds of delights. Now, the second prince had a weakness for the pleasures of the flesh, so he didn't think too long before accepting the offer. But no sooner had he flung himself expectantly onto her bed than the bed turned over, dumping him into an underground prison. In the dungeon, he found a number of other young suitors who had met a similar fate. That was the end of the road for the second son and he never returned home.

More time passed and eventually the third son, who was thought to be the dumbling of the family, was ready to go out into the world. The king, who had now lost two sons, was hesitant to let his youngest go and the boy had to beg his father to allow him to leave.

Eventually, the king relented and gave him a horse and he was on his way. He soon came to the signpost and had to decide which of the three directions he would choose—hunger for his horse, hunger for himself, or the third route which promised only death.

Now, the third son knew that his older brothers had tried the roads to the left and to the right; and he knew that both had failed. He therefore chose the road straight ahead, realizing that he had no other option than to risk death.

By and by, he came to a house on the side of the road in which lived a witch called Baba Yaga. The witch invited the young boy in and sat him down, as if to make him comfortable. And when she thought she had him off-guard, she popped the question which she believed would destroy him.

"Tell me," she said in an innocent tone, "did you come here by choice, or did you have to come?"

The prince, understanding that there was no rational answer to her either/or question, saw the trap and refused to answer replying merely, "Shut up woman and give me something to eat!"

The unexpected retort broke the power inherent in the paradoxical question and with it the witch's power. The next day, the prince continued on his way and had many adventures. Many years later, he returned to his kingdom a changed man, fully matured and ready to assume the responsibilities of being a king.

What does such a story have to tell us? Beyond their function as childhood entertainment, fairy tales often attempt to teach those sorts of lessons which cannot be otherwise imparted. Their method is experiential; and their content secondarily refers to the unfolding of our inner potential and the expression of our spirit in its fullness. Joseph Campbell and a growing number of others have written extensively about the power of myth in our lives, relating the common themes running through the mythological stories of various cultures.

This particular Russian story has all the marks of a childhood fairy tale, with a king, various princes and a witch. But it also tells the story of the choices which we face in life. We are all looking for the perfect situation, the perfect spouse, or the job which will provide security and happiness, but life has a habit of placing us in situations which are not quite as clear-cut as the choices offered on the signpost.

Let's start our analysis of the myth by defining the meaning of the primary symbols. In this situation, the king might represent the conscious self, and/or the prevailing cultural consciousness. The three princes represent three different temperaments which will deal differently with choices in life.

Each of the princes rides a horse. The rider can be said to represent the intellect or rational mind, which controls and directs our actions; and the horse, our feeling or irrational side. Horse and rider come to a signpost which forces a choice. The first option is to plentifully nourish the intellect at the expense of the emotions.

INTELLECT-DOMINANT SOLUTIONS

To identify ourselves with our rational minds is a choice many of us make in our lives, allowing our intellects to decide what job to go for, what person to marry, how to spend Saturday evening or where to holiday. Feelings are often thought inappropriate or downright dangerous, and so are suppressed. This kind of existence is normally marked by a nearly unquestioning adherence to various rules—either personally or culturally defined—the absence of which leaves the intellect floundering and insecure.

"Without rules of civilized behaviour man would descend into a state of anarchy"—such maxims have always justified the existence of laws which govern society, and the need to suppress feeling is taken pretty much for granted. Take, for example, a situation in which we are pulled over to the side of the road by a policeman for some minor infringement of the rules of the road. Feeling might prompt us to punch the policeman in the nose, but rational thought would probably contradict the urge, since the consequences of challenging authority are not usually acceptable.

In most such cases, intellect overrules feeling with the result that many people live lives of quiet desperation—in soul-destroying jobs, or damaged marriages, living the struggle between their emotional and rational natures—in the belief that change is not possible. For many of us, the pressure to produce a paycheque which covers our various financial commitments outweighs our desire to embark on a different course. We may have been brought up to believe that life is tough, that it is not always possible to have what we want, or that it is only right to sacrifice ourselves for the sake of the family. The rules will differ depending on the culture we were brought up in, or the values passed on to us by our parents, but it is almost certain that rules there will be.

Starving our emotional nature long enough brings us to an impasse—an emotional and conceptual rigidity which leaves us vulnerable to accident and illness. In the myth, that susceptibility is represented by the snake which the first prince finds after his horse has given up. He takes the snake home only to have it angrily rejected by his father, the king.

We have seen numerous people who seem to fit the pattern. The stresses of life, work, and relationships build up to the point where something has to give, and for many people in our car-oriented society, an automobile accident may intervene. This is not to say that accidents are not accidents, but it is possible that there is more to them than meets the eye. After all, when we are under a lot of stress, we are more likely to have an accident, any accident, and a typical doctor's day will involve more stress-related illnesses than anything else.

In the case of the accident then, the snake which the prince picks up might stand for the chronic pain which often follows a motor vehicle accident; and in the case of illness, the stigma attached to people judged unable to cope with life. In either case, the individual must carry the problem around until a resolution is found.

For many people this is quite a problem, because no resolution is forthcoming. In the myth, the prince takes the snake back to the king, but the king is so angry that he puts him in prison—as though trying to make his problem son go away. Similarly, a doctor will try to "kill the pain," or "get rid of" a patient's illness.

Now, in many traditions, the snake represents paradox—mysterious and evil, but of enormous benefit. In the

Hippocratic tradition, the Aesculapian staff is entwined by two snakes representing the power of healing. So our prince in picking up the snake may have sensed in its healing power the possibility of getting his life back on track.

It is highly significant that the king is unable to see the snake's potential value. Similarly, the medical profession, in its attempt to "kill" chronic pain may be unable to see the potential for true healing contained within that pain. As a result, like the king, we may write off patients with functional illnesses as unfit to rule their kingdoms, and imprison them in a life of dependence on the medical profession. In doing so, we inadvertently do a great disservice by denying people the opportunity to learn the lesson the snake has to offer.

EMOTION-DOMINANT SOLUTIONS

Now what about the left-hand path? That is the path which attracts unrestrainedly emotional individuals whose lives are guided by feeling to the detriment of the intellect. Though this is perhaps a less common path than the intellect-dominant one, many people feel inclined to sensuality as a reaction to the entrapment and rigidity they experience in their day-to-day existence. The youth movement of the sixties is an example of this enacted on a large scale. Spouses who indulge in love affairs or drink in order to deal with their marital problems are feeding their emotional natures, trying to recover a balance lost.

Uncontrolled sensuality creates an impasse of a different kind. In the myth, the second prince is enticed into a stranger's bed and falls into a dungeon from which there is no escape. To be lost in one's sexuality, in alcohol, or drugs is indeed to be in prison—and the second prince never returns.

THE THIRD CHOICE

Unlike the first two, the third prince has to beg to be allowed to go on the quest; and when he arrives at the signpost, he chooses to die. That alarming choice is not really a choice at all. Most of us can see only the choice between rationality and feeling—both of which have their limitations. The third option is not even considered. It appears so absolute that no one would consciously make it unless there were no other choice. In other words, only when we are in a position where death is certain does "choosing" death become an option.

This is certainly true in a physical sense—if we are terminally ill, we might choose to hasten death. This story, however, can be read as referring to psychological death. We can choose to die to our illusions about life, and simply get on with living.

The chronically ill eventually reach a point where they know they have lost everything. The hope of a quick recovery fades as therapies and treatments prove ineffectual. The person's employment may be on the line, since work may be difficult or impossible; and physicians, family, friends and insurance agents begin to suspect a malingerer. Marriage partners under such stress often threaten to leave, and children have trouble understanding their parents' mysterious limitations.

It is out of such desperate situations that the will to try the third path may come. Personal annihilation seems all but accomplished anyway, what's the difference? The third choice is a choice of no choice: the point where there seems no glimmer of hope left either rationally or emotionally. It is the place from which a paradox emerges and may be solved.

In retrospect, illness may be seen as a necessary preliminary to making the decision to live or to die—just as the third prince chose the road to death because he knew the other two led to disaster. When Baba Yaga, the witch, poses him the question, "Did you come this way by choice or not?" the prince cannot answer as either possible response would be both true and false. Attempting to answer would have entangled him intellectually and denied the paradox he had chosen. The witch's question is designed to ensnare the unwary traveller in a dilemma, thereby allowing her to establish her power.

Had that occurred, the prince would never have escaped alive. In making the choice to take the third path, the prince decided to let go of his intellect, understanding that a paradox cannot be "solved." Similarly, we cannot make the choice to die psychologically unless we have struggled long enough to come to the witch's house knowing there is no logical solution—that the only answer is no answer at all, but to get on with the situation at hand. In the circumstances of the story it was time to eat. The third path, therefore, is the path of transformation, a path we want to explore in this book.

Chapter Two

THE WOMAN
WITHOUT HANDS

To listen is not to hear, to look is not to see

Our first story illustrates some of the intellectual dilemmas to which our psyche may be prone. Now we come to another and different story illustrating the challenges to its emotional aspect.

There was once a miller who neglected his mill and so was reduced to cutting firewood in the forest to make his living. One day, he chanced upon an ugly dwarf who asked him what he was doing, whereupon the miller told his sorry tale. The dwarf offered to make him rich and successful in return for no more than whatever was to be found in the garden behind the mill.

The miller quickly agreed, thinking that the garden contained nothing but an old apple tree, and the dwarf went on his way. The miller returned home and, sure enough, the money started to roll in.

The miller and his wife had three years in which to enjoy their new-found wealth before the dwarf returned to demand his startling fee. Unbeknownst to her father, the miller's only daughter—by now a lovely young woman—happened to have been playing in the garden at the time of their original bargain. It was she that the dwarf had come for. When the miller appeared reluctant, the dwarf threatened to take him away instead, and the man eventually saw that he had little choice, and reluctantly agreed to honour their contract.

As it happened however, the young girl was listening to what was going on and invoked the help of her guardian spirit. On the advice of her protector, she washed herself carefully, so that when the dwarf returned he was not able to take her. He angrily instructed the miller to make sure that she didn't wash again, and said that he would be back for her the next day.

That evening the miller locked his daughter in her room so that she couldn't bathe. She was very frightened and prayed again for assistance from her guardian spirit. When no help appeared forthcoming, she began to cry from the depths of her soul. Soon there were tears pouring down her face, forming rivers of water which washed her clean; and again the dwarf could not take her. In a rage, the little man told the miller to chop off the girl's hands so she couldn't pray again, and when the miller balked at such a gruesome task, again threatened to take him instead.

Reluctantly, the miller went to his daughter and with some misgivings explained to her what he had to do. She submitted to her father's wishes and held out her hands to be severed. That night she felt the helplessness of abandonment, and tears poured from her eyes like a waterfall, washing all the blood away, thwarting the dwarf for the third and last time.

With the dwarf out of the way, the miller regained his composure, promising his daughter that he would do anything for her and look after her for the rest of her life. By this time, however, the mutilated and betrayed daughter found it hard to trust her father's sincerity. She decided that she must leave home and live on her own, despite the fact that the dwarf had put a parting curse on her leaving her unable to speak. So she bound her wounds and wandered alone out into the world with no one but her guardian spirit to protect her.

By and by she came to a garden in which there was a pear tree; being hungry but without hands to hold the fruit, she ate a pear as it hung off the tree. She found it quite tasty and so returned on successive nights, when the garden appeared empty, to nibble at the fruit.

Now, it so happened that the garden belonged to the king and he was very angry when he found that someone was stealing his pears. He set the gardener to watch, and the following night when she came, the gardener was amazed to see a beautiful young woman eating a pear without using her hands. Because of her peculiar behaviour, the gardener decided to inform the king directly rather than accosting her, and on hearing his story the king was so intrigued that he decided to stand watch himself the next night.

Overcome at the sight of the mysterious woman, the king invited her to his palace; and despite her inability to speak to him, the king fell in love with her and made her his queen. And in order that she might appear in public, he had the royal silversmith make her a pair of silver hands.

Time went by, and the birth of the couple's first child was imminent. As the king had to be away on affairs of state, he asked his mother to be sure to tell him the outcome of the birth. Not long after, the mute queen delivered a healthy young prince and everyone in the royal household was overjoyed. The king's mother sent off the glad tidings to the king, but the wicked dwarf, who had been biding his time, bewitched the messenger and changed the message to read that the young queen had given birth to a changeling.

The king was distraught at the news, but couldn't believe that his beloved queen was a witch. He sent back a message to his mother to look after the queen but to get rid of the changeling. Again the dwarf changed the message, so that it read as an order to kill both queen and child, and to save the young woman's eyes and tongue as proof that the deed had been done.

The old queen was dumbfounded at the unexpected response and didn't know what to do. Eventually, she decided to use a slaughtered calf's eyes and tongue to show the king when he returned, and to warn the queen to take her infant and go into hiding. And so the outcast queen, betrayed for a second time, took her newborn son and wandered into the forest again with only her guardian spirit to protect her.

The young mother eventually found a small hut in the forest where she decided to live and bring up her son, and there she eked out a meager existence. One day, while the unfortunate queen was out walking in the wood with her baby on her back, she came across a spring, and as she bent to get a drink, the infant tumbled from her back and fell into the water. In the shock of the moment, she instinctively reached out the stubs of her arms to save him, and as her arms plunged into the water her hands reappeared, as good as new.

The king meanwhile had returned to his palace, and was devastated to be presented with the tongue and eyes of his beloved. When he at last heard the true story, he set out at once to find his wife and child and to make amends. But it took seven years of intense searching before he came across her cottage in the woods; and by then it had been so long that he didn't recognize the woman he saw there, let alone the seven-year old child who was with her. Eventually, by showing him her old pair of silver hands, she convinced him that she really was his queen and that the boy was his son. The king was ecstatic, and all three returned to the palace to live happily ever after.

Our emotional nature has different problems than our rational nature. Mythologically, stories concerning our emotional nature present quests of introspection in isolation rather than worldly adventure and conquest, quests having to do with *being* rather than with *doing*. And although our culture has in the past often associated the emotional with the female, and the rational with the male, each of us possesses both aspects, and it is important for us not to fall into the trap of gender-typing them in such a way as to deny their real meaning.

The story of the miller's daughter suggests that our emotional natures have to deal with problems of paralysis of personal power. What does it mean to say that our feelings have become paralyzed? How can the myth help us to see how we can regain our personal power?

Let's start by defining some of the terms in the story. Say that the miller is a father figure; and the dwarf is the power of negativity, a negativity driven by a need for power and security—a drive itself often motivated by a deep-seated fear of annihilation. Recognizing the dwarf as representative of negative forces is not identical to judging him bad—mythologically, good and evil are determined by the way we react to the challenges they pose.

If the king—who has authority over the actions of everyone in the story but the dwarf—represents the conscious intellect, which controls feeling, the silver hands might represent our coping mechanisms. Such mechanisms allow us to "carry on" without having to acknowledge our mutilations.

DISEMPOWERMENT AND EMOTIONAL WOUNDING

As the miller was often the richest merchant in a village, that our miller is said to be poor suggests that he is not very good at being a miller. More than that, he seems a startlingly poor father—the story illustrates his willingness to sacrifice his own daughter to make up for his ineptitude as a miller and to bolster his own sense of security.

Such a family relationship is, unfortunately, not uncommon. Many parents unconsciously disempower their children to bolster their own self-worth and to hide their inadequacies; in violent situations this degradation may take the form of physical or sexual abuse. As is now becoming apparent, it is not unusual for children to be sexually abused by members of their family, or other adults.

"Spare the rod and spoil the child" continues to shape our thinking; and child abuse beyond simple discipline is epidemic. Those children who are not actually physically abused, who on the contrary are given every material comfort, may be emotionally starved instead, so that few children reach adulthood unscathed.

As a small child is totally dependent on her parents, her only mechanism for handling such an experience is denial. The rational self has injured the emotional self, and the emotional side can't say so. Each of our own childhoods might provide numerous parallel situations—situations in which our feelings were suppressed for fear of their consequences. In our story, however, feeling doesn't give in to pressure at all easily. On three separate occasions the miller's daughter defies the dwarf's demands by appealing to her inner guide; and by her very outpouring of feeling, her tears, makes her possession by the dwarf impossible. Her strength lies in her faith in her intuition.

At the same time, she gives up her hands to her father. The sacrifice represents the damage done to the child who apparently relinquishes her right to realize her full potential and her ability to operate independently without protest. The emotional being is crippled by giving over its autonomy to the intellect.

THE CURSE OF SILENCE

Our inability to engage our emotional nature leaves us less than whole, and rationality excuses our disability by intimating that control of feelings is the normal way to live. How often have we been admonished not to show our feelings? How often have we been ridiculed for expressing them? For many of us the answer is too often to count, so often in fact that we eventually decide never to show our feelings again. Ultimately, we reach a point where we forget that we were suppressing anything.

Such is the curse of silence: at a certain point we are no longer able to express the essence of our problem. An injury, after all, that begins at a time when we are too small to understand what is happening to us is so deeply buried by the time we reach an age when we could grasp it intellectually that what voice it had has been silenced—by the time she leaves her father's house, the miller's daughter is mute to the world.

SILVER HANDS AND GARBLED MESSAGES

In our story, the king is strangely drawn to the mute and handless woman he observes eating pears in his garden; a choice is made on the basis of feeling, resulting in a marriage between feeling and intellect.

The story suggests that we are often attracted to a career or relationship in which we intuitively feel we may mend our own damaged or missing part. People who go into the healing professions often do so because they want to heal themselves. A man who feels unable to express his emotions may be attracted to an emotionally expressive woman. We are all attracted to something which represents the part of us which is damaged, whatever that may be.

In the myth, the king makes a pair of silver hands for his new queen. The hands allow her to cope with life for the time being: to appear in public, and to fulfil her official duties, but of course they are a bizarre substitute for the real thing. In life, we find that our career, our relationship, or whatever we have chosen to complete ourselves may become our silver hands, allowing us to cope, but without resolving the injury. That is a longer and more solitary task.

The king and queen in the myth produce a child. The promise traditionally represented by the birth of a new baby is that of integration, wholeness and healing within us; of healing in ourselves through our relationships, and our chosen careers. But though the king leaves word for his mother to keep him informed about the birth of his child, the distance between intellect and feeling has become sufficiently wide that the message he gets is garbled and threatens instead of confirming his relationship.

MIND AND BODY; ILLNESS AND HEALTH

What is the origin and consequence of distorted messages? We believe that the "distortion of messages" stage is the critical moment when illness manifests itself.

'Feeling sends desperate messages to the intellect in the form of symptoms, which are attempts on the part of feeling to communicate in the relationship, and to induce the return to wholeness. If the dwarf, who represents a negative force, succeeds in altering the message so that communication is garbled, further symptoms or an illness may emerge.

Migraines, stomach aches, ulcers, hypertension, anxiety, panic attacks, depression, back pain, or almost anything else—a whole panoply of stress-related symptoms may surface, urging us to take a look at what is going on in our lives and to attend to our rational/emotional balance. The body is making a stab at communication, but the intellect gets an entirely different message. Symptoms are read as bad: the king hears that his offspring is a changeling; he is shocked and sends back orders to kill the baby.

Significantly, however, he does not order his wife killed—we wish to kill the symptom of which we are now aware, but want to spare feeling itself, because some part of us recognizes its importance. It is only when the message gets garbled again, that the attempt to kill feeling itself occurs—when our physical symptoms become so threatening that we are willing to injure ourselves in order to get some relief.

Because it doesn't realize the significance of the message-symptoms, and has misinterpreted these messages from the body as bad, the intellect reasons that there is no other option, and the order to "kill" feeling goes out. Fortunately, our emotional side is rarely completely destroyed, it simply goes into hiding—the queen goes off with her child and lives in the woods alone; and the king is left to return home when he is ready.

In life, it seems that our emotional nature often has to go into hiding to mature in isolation until it is capable of full expression. The evolution can either occur slowly over time, or suddenly in a crisis. Typically, the crisis is an illness which seems without effective treatment, or an equivalent event, such as a marriage break-up, or loss of a job. A situation comes along which defies a rational solution and leaves us on the horns of a dilemma. Wholeness, represented by the baby, becomes so threatened that feeling must act quickly and decisively. At that point its real hands grow back; we find our personal power.

The king eventually returns to find his wife and child gone from the palace. When he finds out what he has done, he is distraught and goes on a search for his loved ones. It is the crisis of illness which often brings the intellect to an awareness that something important is missing. The thought "is this all there is?" will often set us on a quest to find what we have lost.

Of course, we may have no idea what we are looking for—as the king does not recognize his wife and child when he sees them, so we do not recognize or validate feeling. We look but we don't see, because we are looking with our mind, and feeling must be experienced in order to be known. It is only when the queen shows the king the silver hands he gave her that he recognizes her.

To know feeling we must relive our pain. It is a most difficult lesson. Healing involves our being in continuous interaction with feeling, which results from a willingness to live with the pain of our childhood wound, *every day*. Healing is not something which happens and which can then be forgotten. Wholeness is a way of living.

When the connection is made between intellect and feeling, the process of healing begins. When their meaning in the context of our lives becomes clear, migraines disappear, stomach upsets settle down, and chest pains diminish. Clear messages finally impinge on our conscious awareness. Feeling unites with the intellect and the wholeness of the relationship, represented by the reunion of the king, the queen and their growing child, is re-established.

Chapter Three

THE ILLUSION OF OBJECTIVITY

Science is not science; objectivity is subjective

$\mathcal{T}$wo thousand years ago, a Cretan sage named Menedis devised a statement that has since become synonymous with the word paradox in the West. That statement was, "All Cretans are liars." If the statement was true, it made Menedis—who was Cretan—a liar, which made his statement false—Cretans were not liars—which meant that his statement was true again, which made him again a liar. That paradox leaves us in the difficult position of having to entertain a statement as both true and not true at the same time.

The essence of life is paradox. When we try to pin it down we get into trouble. The cell membrane shouldn't be, but is; the universe itself has no rational explanation for its existence. Life shouldn't be, but is.

Western science attempts to deny the paradox of life and to make it manageable and controllable by allowing as truth only what it understands as "objective" evidence. The practice was developed with the best of intentions, but the essential paradox remains and humankind's continuing efforts to deny the mystery of existence is causing more and more problems.

Conventional medicine is a system of medicine which is based on the scientific method. We live in a culture founded on the validity of science, and one in which few have questioned whether that validity has limits.

In fact, orthodox science has major limitations. It arises from cultural assumptions—such as the possibility of objectivity—that have been shown, over the past eighty years or so, to be inadequate.

And yet we as a culture press blindly ahead in our everyday lives as if those assumptions were absolutely true. Science has become the silver hands of our culture. We have all accepted objectivity as the only standard of the scientific method. A premise based on such false assumptions must eventually give us false conclusions, as the distortion introduced at the start becomes magnified in each link in the chain of logic. The end result could be a significant and possibly disastrous deviation from truth.

In short, a small error at the beginning will, if uncorrected, produce a large error at the end. And as the culture goes, so goes our medicine, so go our diseases. To understand the paradox of our medicine and of our cultural illness, we must grasp the assumptions on which we base our lives. We must understand the fundamental error implicit in the practice of objective scientific enquiry, an error which has by now become all-embracing in its implications.

When the analysis has been made, we can perhaps begin to see how the correction of such a fundamental error in our thinking may lead us to very different conclusions. We can come to see that, like the characters in our first two stories, medicine itself must risk everything before it can live again.

THE CARTESIAN SYSTEM OF THOUGHT

Our present assumptions about scientific thinking date back to the time of René Descartes (1596-1650). At the age of 23, he had an intuition which led to the publication of his famous essay, "Discourse on Method."

The essay contains three tenets which have over time become the fundamental building blocks of our modern scientific culture. They are: the certainty of scientific knowledge;

the separation of mind and matter; and the universe as machine. Let's look at these tenets in turn.

1. THE CERTAINTY OF SCIENTIFIC KNOWLEDGE

We understand scientific knowledge as objective knowledge, and objectivity as the basis of all legitimate scientific enquiry. Eliminating as far as is possible the observer, science attempts to define the observed through reproducible experiments. Knowledge gained in this way is considered to be real. Take, for example, drug trials. Whenever a new treatment or a new drug is being tested, observer bias is said to be ruled out by "double-blinding"—that is, neither the patient (single-blind) nor the doctor (double-blind) knows whether the test drug or a placebo is being administered.

Medical research which does not observe such principles of objectivity is regarded as second-rate. Pick up any respectable medical journal; it will contain reports of objective, double-blind studies, and would consider no other research acceptable for publication. Yet if we look closely, we will see that by insisting on objective criteria, medical science demonstrates a shocking disregard for the discoveries of modern physics and the quantum reality that that physics describes. In other words, an error which crept in to our understanding of the disease process many years ago still stubbornly persists in spite of well-founded discoveries in the very field which medicine purports to base its research procedures on: science.

The truth is that in most fields the kind of science which aims at objectivity is no longer deemed scientific; modern scientific enquiry has had to acknowledge that the world cannot be observed or defined in the absence of an observer; and that in fact without the observer there might be said to be no reality.

The function of the observer was brought home forcibly to physicists in the early part of the century when they were trying to grapple with the paradox of wave-particle duality which was cropping up in their observations of the nature of sub-microscopic particles. Albert Einstein in an experiment involving "black body" radiation had proposed, among other things, that light waves had both a wave-like nature and a particle-like nature.

His proposal seemed absurd at the time—how could something behave as both a wave and a particle at once?—yet it was sound. Scientists who struggled with the problem over the next twenty years came up with an even more startling observation: when they structured the experiment to show that matter is wave-like, then matter appeared wave-like. If, on the other hand, they structured the experiment to show it to be particle-like then, paradoxically, it appeared particulate.

In other words, reality is observer-dependent—what is seen depends on who is seeing; there is no such thing as objectivity. But despite the fact that this is now thoroughly accepted by physicists, it has not seemed to have had much impact on modern scientific medicine.

The reason is hard to fathom. Perhaps it is assumed that what is true for the microscopic world need not apply in the macroscopic world. The argument has certainly been made that what is known as an "averaging of quantum randomness"—a process which produces an identifiable macroscopic world—allows us to treat the macroscopic world as if it were composed of separate objects.

Though the argument is attractive and is valid up to a point, it is dangerous because it allows us to persist in accepting a severely limited view of the world as "scientific." Consider a rose. Everyone knows that roses are often red, and we would all agree that for our everyday purposes an acceptable answer to the question, "What colour is this rose?" could be, "The rose is red." But is it a "true" statement in an absolute sense? Given that humans can see the red end of the light spectrum and bees cannot, a bee looking at the rose in question will see it differently. To the question, "What colour is this rose?" then, the real answer must always be, "It depends on who is looking."

What appears to be an objective statement is actually *a statement of collective agreement* among observers concerning the commonality of their subjective experience. Thus, the so-called "objective" stance, championed so enthusiastically by traditional scientific medicine, is really just a cover-up for a "subjective" stance, a stance which attempts to separate and dissect things which cannot ultimately be separated or dissected. Furthermore, in spite of the fact that the subject-object division is an untenable proposition, modern medicine persists in choosing to invalidate subjective experience in favour of what it conceives of as objective—with disastrous results.

2. MIND AND MATTER ARE SEPARATE

The second tenet of Cartesian thinking is that mind and matter are separate. That proposition has led to the idea that physical illnesses are of the body, and mental illnesses are in the mind, and that there is not much connection between the two. This has led to the separation of physical medicine and psychiatry, to the extent that psychiatric hospitals are actually geographically separate from the main part of many hospitals.

This mind-body split also led to medical reductionism—the notion that the body can best be understood by breaking it down into its constituent parts. Reductionism is the impetus for our belief that the "best" doctors are those who specialize in only one aspect of the body, and physicians who treat the body as a whole unit, the general practitioners, are less knowledgeable. Unfortunately, today's general practitioners are also so schooled in reductionism that those few who are inclined to think holistically have usually achieved that understanding through experience rather than training.

But the idea of a mind-body separation is only an approximation, a way of thinking designed to be consistent with the stance of scientific objectivity. Even a cursory examination of the proposition will reveal an obvious contradiction. The paradox is that even if the body and mind were separate, they would not be separate.

Chronic depression is known to depress the immune system, and therefore set the stage for physical disease, ranging from catching a simple cold to cancer; and recent experiments in psycho-neuro-immunology have confirmed the intimate connection between the nervous system and the immune system and vice versa, documenting the ability of certain cells in the immune system to produce neuro-transmitters. It is also commonly observed that this mind-body connection works in reverse—a patient with physical pain will become depressed if that pain goes on long enough. In short, any disease which affects the body will also affect the mind, and what affects the mind also affects the body.

The apparent separation of mind and matter is therefore just the result of a preconception—what might be called a cultural superstition—endemic in Western cultures after the so-called "Enlightenment," which Descartes' ideas helped to fuel. In reality it simply does not exist.

Yet despite the fact that evidence for the mind-body connection is coming from respectable scientists using standard objective criteria, the idea is strongly resisted by orthodox medicine. We still behave as if physical diseases are somehow more real than mental disease, and feel unjustly accused if a physician suggests that the cause of an illness might lie in the mind. But the fact is that all diseases have a physical, mental, emotional, spiritual, and environmental aspect. And to begin to see the connection between mind and body is to begin to see the connection between all aspects of ourselves, and of ourselves and the universe.

A more sinister aspect of our denial of such connectedness is the traditional separation of individual from disease. In our culture, disease is seen as an entity separate from the individual, an alien invader to be fought and destroyed. And while the approach works well for infectious diseases such as tuberculosis or staphylococcal pneumonia, it simply does not work for the vast majority of illnesses confronting the modern-day physician: illnesses ranging from anxiety to cancer.

Modern physics tells us that reality is best described as an indivisible whole, that everything is related to everything else, and yet modern medicine persists in separating mind from body, body from disease.

Just as the mind and body are connected, so in fact are body and disease allied. From that perspective the idea that disease should be eradicated is absurd. *Disease is fundamentally an extension of the self.*

3. THE UNIVERSE IS A MACHINE

The third tenet of Cartesian thinking is that the universe is a machine—rather like a clock, which is wound up, and which will run until it has no more energy left. Machines are generally designed to perform kinetically to achieve certain tasks, so that:

$$A \quad causes \quad B \quad causes \quad C$$

The notion of cause and effect is fundamental to traditional scientific enquiry. Diseases, too, are assumed to have particular causes, whether or not any cause can be found. There is a commonly accepted assumption among physicians and public alike that science will eventually discover causes for every disease.

Once again, such a view may be predicated on a limited and outdated understanding. Modern physics has recognized linear cause and effect as a limited concept in a universe perceived as an indivisible whole, infinitely correlated. In such a universe, everything or nothing is the cause of everything else. There is literally no specific cause for anything—everything arises at the same time. In order to present that notion in a linear way we are forced to describe a circular model in which:

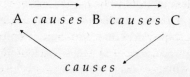

This, of course, is a paradoxical expression which really questions the validity of the model itself. However, rather than give up the linear model of cause and effect, medical science has invented the concept of the "feedback loop." The theory allows scientists to maintain the illusion of cause and effect, so that the basic assumption does not have to be questioned.

In the feedback loop:

A causes B causes C which feeds back to affect A either positively or negatively.

The central difficulty with the feedback loop is that it contradicts the implicit linearity of the cause and effect model with respect to the passage of time. Since cause must precede effect *in time*, the model only creates a paradox when the feedback loop is introduced. Simply put, C cannot feedback to A if C does not exist prior to A in time. Unlike machines which may be designed in linear ways, the A, B, and C of biological systems all arise at the same time, and the difference between the systems clearly throws open the whole question of cause and effect, making the model of the feedback loop untenable in biological sciences.

Yet so strong is our belief in cause and effect that it is virtually impossible for medical science, patients or their doctors to give it up. Patients want to know what caused their illness, and doctors want to give them a plausible explanation. Yet often there is no particular cause of an illness apart from the patient. The patient, embedded in the fabric of society and the universe, *is* the illness—the cause is its effect.

Experienced physicians are often intuitively aware of the difficulty posed by "cause" but find themselves in a very difficult position if they try to point it out. Not only do physicians face vigorous denial if they dare to suggest no cause—most patients would rather be given a "culprit" than accept personal responsibility for their health—but more importantly, the idea of "no cause" poses a challenge to the doctor-patient relationship, and might even be seen to question the relationship itself.

Even when there seems to be a manifest "cause" for a disease, closer analysis may reveal a conceptual flaw in assuming a cause-and-effect continuum. Let's take the example of streptococcal pharyngitis, a common enough disease normally treated with penicillin. Few would argue that the streptococcus is not the cause of the pharyngitis, but studies have shown that some twenty percent of the population carry streptococcus in the throat and nasal passages without any deleterious effect, while only a handful of people actually get the disease. Clearly there are other factors. In other words, streptococcus is not the cause, but merely one factor amongst others necessary for the disease to express itself.

To say that the streptococci cause pharyngitis is much the same as arguing that traffic causes traffic accidents. Clearly, certain elements are necessary factors, but they are not *causes* in a linear sense. Though the streptococcus might still be considered causal in that it is the most significant of the complex of factors, the factor far outstripping all others as "cause," are the patients themselves.

Because it requires the physician to confront the patient however, that factor is normally overlooked. It is far easier to treat pharyngitis with penicillin than to confront patients with their personal responsibility—especially when penicillin works so well!

The limitations of contemporary scientific thought leave our reasoning floundering for a more acceptable conceptual framework to explain illness. If science cannot show us the truth about reality, then what can?

Chapter Four

FINDING ANOTHER PERSPECTIVE

One point of view deserves another

It is not easy to just invent a different philosophical basis for medicine. If it were, the alternate system would probably already be around. It is because we have no experience of another system that we must discover such a system by inference. With different systems of thought, there is a fundamental problem of perception to be overcome, which can be illustrated by a simple analogy. If two people were talking to each other about a dollar bill, and they had each seen the dollar bill from opposite sides, then they could be forgiven for thinking that they were talking about two substantially different objects.

Though both are describing the same bill, neither would recognize the other's description and each would be convinced that his or her own description was correct. Unless we agree that it is possible to turn the bill over and look at it from the other side, we will remain unconvinced of another's point of view. Similarly, when it comes to describing reality, we must first admit there may be another perspective before we will be able to consider shifting our own point of view.

Shifting our perspective can be especially difficult, however, given such a large concept as reality. The view we currently hold is usually that of a collective consciousness, or prevailing cultural mind-set; and that being the case there may be no one to indicate the opposite view. If everyone agreed on the description of the dollar bill, there would be no reason to suppose that there might be another way of looking at it.

If we take the dollar bill and begin to turn it over slowly it will at one point nearly disappear, or at least becomes a very thin line. That point has been referred to in many ways: point of dissolution, point of nothingness, point of phase transition, etc. Each of the terms attempts to describe a state of being between two other states and this point of phase transition has a certain magical quality to it. It represents the letting go of the old and the anticipation of the new. In life, the experience may look and feel like annihilation.

INFERRING THE OPPOSITE PERSPECTIVE

By defining medicine's traditional perspective using the Cartesian model, we can infer the existence of a paradoxical opposite. These assumptions permeate Western society and form the modus operandi of conventional medicine. They have led to our belief in rationalism, causality, objectivity, and the separation of medicine and psychiatry. The assumptions work very well in acute emergency situations, but are limited when illness becomes chronic. By listing the assumptions on the left-hand side of the page, we can infer their paradoxical opposite assumptions in the opposite column (fig. 1).

When we make the lists we find that we have defined what seems a very strange outlook on our existence. However, on closer examination it becomes apparent that we are not actually doing anything new at all, because what we have done is to stumble into the subject of dialectics, a subject which is at the very root of other more traditional forms of medicine.

In particular, dialectics form the philosophical base of Traditional Chinese Medicine (TCM), which is at least five thousand years old. The ideas of yin and yang—paradoxical opposites—fit into Figure 1 with consummate ease. What is more, Cartesian thinking can be classified broadly as yang, and its inferred opposite as yin. Chinese philosophical thought can therefore be seen to be inclusive of Western thought, while Western thought has no way of incorporating Chinese holistic thinking.

· BIOMEDICAL PERSPECTIVE	· INFERRED OPPOSITE
· objective	· subjective
· cause and effect	· acausal (without cause)
· mind and matter separate	· mind and matter connected
· structural	· functional
· logical/rational	· intuitive
· separate	· connected

Fig. 1—The biomedical perspective and its inferred opposite.

Given our collective perspective, it is not surprising that many respected scientists have tried to explain the workings of Chinese medicine by means of conventional scientific analysis. The fact that objective analysis is not the right tool to unlock the mysteries of TCM is not usually considered, and the conventional wisdom blindly writes off Chinese philosophy as irrelevant to the West. It is argued that because Chinese thinking is ancient, it must be primitive and outmoded—a product of childish thinking. It never occurs to us that the reverse might be the truth.

In fact, Chinese philosophy is based on functional rather than on structural analysis. In place of objectivity, it substitutes subjective experience or "feeling." Rather than seeing illness as separate, it sees illness as an aspect of the self. And instead of dealing in linear time and notions of "cause," it sees a pattern of disharmony existing in an individual in the present moment.

In conventional medicine, we regularly come across patients who have illnesses with no known cause, where the primary problem is difficult to pin down. We actually describe these patients as "functional," using the very word which should suggest an alternative approach, yet often missing the opportunity provided to explore that approach. By using the word "functional," we usually imply that the patient is neurotic and needs the services of a psychiatrist, rather than question the validity of our conventional viewpoint and look for a different model.

Traditional Chinese Medicine, as it happens, is a system of medicine based on functional analysis and on feeling, thereby conveniently filling a gap in our thinking. TCM complements conventional medical wisdom as its inferred opposite perspective, providing an approach based on the other side of the dollar bill. Felix Mann describes how "feeling" forms the basis of Chinese medicine in the following words:

> Much of Chinese medical theory describes what the patient feels. The patient feels differences in energy. He feels something along the course of meridians. The Western doctor often excludes the patient's feelings and measures serum electrolytes, haemoglobin and faecal fat instead.

The strength of conventional medicine lies in the fact that when the haemoglobin is low, rational treatment may be prescribed. However, more often than not, people feel ill without any noticeable change in blood chemistry, leaving the doctor without any rational basis for treating them. In that case the doctor has little choice but to send the patient home, or else to initiate further laboratory investigations at great expense. Either way the conventional medical approach often leaves both parties feeling frustrated.

No conceptual framework exists in the West which allows a therapeutic approach based on feelings alone. Conventional medicine tries to look after the body only, and leaves psychiatry to look after problems of the mind. When traditional Western physicians cannot find anything wrong physiologically, they have no choice but to deny their patients' experience of illness, invalidating them rather than medicine itself.

But psychiatry, like medicine, has chosen to view the mind mechanistically as if its functioning were strictly a result of biochemical processes and the "cause" of mental illness, biochemical imbalances. That approach leads to treating mental illnesses with drugs: depression is treated with anti-depressants, and anxiety with tranquilizers. While the approach certainly has some value, for the most part it obscures the fact that the emotional side of the individual is trying to get a message to the intellect. Anxiety and depression are natural responses to life situations, to problems which we think are unsolvable. However, it is precisely those paradoxical situations which could encourage us to choose the third path.

At best, drug treatment merely postpones the time of reckoning, and deprives us of the opportunity to change which is presented by illness. At worst, we create drug dependence and disturb body chemistry without understanding the consequences.

Illness brought about by treatment or therapy is known as iatrogenic, or doctor-induced, and it now accounts for approximately twenty percent of all illnesses. The mechanistic philosophy espoused by conventional medicine has become an increasingly powerful force perpetuating a disease mentality in society. The tranquilizer offers to solve the patient's problem with no effort on his part in the same way that the dwarf solved the miller's need for money. Tranquilizers offer the promise of happiness, but if we take them for an extended period we will eventually become drug-dependent.

The miller had no idea of the consequences of giving the dwarf whatever was in his garden, just as we have no idea what we will forfeit when we ask the doctor for tranquilizers. Unfortunately, very often the doctor has no idea either. Some physicians are aware of the dilemma, but despite their best efforts they find that they have many patients on long-term drug therapy for one reason or another.

As a society, we seem to be incapable of doing anything about the crisis of inappropriate drug use, because the problem of drugs is created by their very availability. What would have happened if the miller had known what was in his garden? That would no doubt have changed everything. Had the miller known his daughter was in the garden, he would in all probability have told the dwarf to leave him alone. But then there would have been no need for the story. If we were brought up in full awareness of the consequences of our decisions, there would be nothing for us to learn in our passage through life.

The story of the miller has applications for us because it is showing us *how we behave*. It is a story about the tragedies and triumphs of our own lives. Such stories contain information we need to transform our limited understanding of the meaning of existence, pointing the way to the other side of the dollar bill.

If we struggle long enough with the discomfort wrought by illness we will eventually turn the dollar bill over and see that another side exists. Other possibilities can then appear which provide the answers we are looking for, and the acquisition of new ways of being and thinking more than compensates for the illness we had to endure; to the point where we may see the illness as the best thing which could have happened.

When we recognize disease as a balancing factor, as the part of our wholeness which has been denied, we are empowered to seek healing through expanding our awareness and looking for alternate concepts and we can simultaneously abandon the effort to eradicate the illness through conventional treatment. Such a total reversal of our approach to illness amounts to what we call a "transformation" of personal philosophy, and the change in attitude is the key element which activates our intrinsic healing system.

Chapter Five

PHASE TRANSITION

Where there is nothing, there is everything

*I*n the last chapter we touched on the notion of the space which lies between two polarized concepts. With the help of the image of a crisp, flat dollar bill slowly turned over, we visualized the point of phase transition—the place between places, the situation between situations—where it seems to disappear. Phase transition, then, is a place of seeming nothingness, and paradoxically, the place of new possibilities.

In order to engage the healing experience, we need to find a way to enter into this experience rather than observe it, to experience it first hand. To reach the place of phase transition, we must be willing to let go of our concept of reality and wait without particular expectations for a new and different experience. We must trust that this new awareness will emerge, because we will never be able to glimpse a new perspective without first letting go of the old one. In other words, we cannot see both sides of the dollar bill at the same time.

Phase transitions are well described in many mythological stories. In these stories, the hero or heroine is commonly required to risk something akin to annihilation, but is rewarded for such fearlessness with undreamed of transformations—their "happily ever after." One of the clearest examples of such transformations is the well known story about the princess and the frog. The princess is put in a situation where she has to kiss a loathsome frog—perhaps the farthest thing she could imagine from her conception of how her life should be. Her reward, however, is new life: the "frog" turns into a handsome prince with whom she lives happily ever after.

SIR GAWAIN AND THE LADY RAGNELL

There is another story of the Knights of the Round Table in which one of the knights, Sir Gawain, is compelled to marry the ugliest of women. The story goes something like this. One day, long ago, King Arthur was out hunting in the woods where he became separated from his party; and very shortly after losing his way, met a knight who made bold to threaten the king's life. Now King Arthur, who considered himself a civilized man, suggested that it would be unchivalrous to kill an unarmed opponent and proposed that instead his assassin devise a wager. The knight obliged him by posing the question, "What is it that women most desire?," demanding that Arthur return in a year with the answer.

The poor king was mystified by the surprising question and asked the help of his loyal friend Sir Gawain; and together the two of them combed the countryside during the ensuing months looking for the answer. Eventually, King Arthur was stopped by an old hag on the road who claimed to be the murderous knight's sister, Lady Ragnell. The mysterious woman told the king that she knew the answer to the riddle, but would only reveal her life-saving knowledge for a price. The desperate monarch promised her anything in his realm, but could barely conceal his horror when the old crone asked for Sir Gawain's hand in marriage. Gawain, on the other hand, hearing the old woman's stipulation, gracefully accepted and unconditionally pledged her his troth.

When the year expired, and Arthur returned to the wood to meet his would-be executioner, he was naturally reluctant to force his trusty Gawain to honour his pledge by using the knowledge the old woman had given them, and so presented all their other ideas first to see if they would satisfy him. The knight, however, sneeringly rejected each in turn and eventually, growing tired of the game, threatened to carry out his original sentence. Seeing no other way out of his dilemma, Arthur finally proffered the answer which the old hag has revealed.

"Women desire their sovereignty," the king declared as the knight raised his sword. The knight was enraged to hear the correct answer at the last moment like that, but held his swing and stalked off leaving Arthur with his head. As the king staggered to his feet and prepared to get out of the woods and back to his castle, the old hag turned up to collect her ransom.

The king acquiesced to the woman's demands, and they returned to the castle to discuss the wedding plans. He suggested the couple marry privately, but Lady Ragnell demanded a big public wedding, shocking all who saw her on the gallant knight's arm with her repulsive appearance and disgusting manners. At the wedding feast she seemed insatiable, eating and drinking everything she could lay her hands on, belching and smacking her lips. But Sir Gawain was not deterred, and after the marriage he escorted her to the bridal chamber where he kissed her and promised to honour their marriage. No sooner had he uttered these words than the hag turned into a beautiful woman.

After the marriage had been consummated, the bride told Sir Gawain that she was only partly liberated from the dreadful curse under which she lived, and that he now would have to choose whether he wanted her beautiful by day and not at night, or beautiful at night but not during the day. It took Gawain only a moment's thought before he answered that either was equally agreeable to him. He had pledged himself, his body, and all his worldly goods to her and therefore she should choose. Once again, as soon as the words were spoken, she was released from the rest of the curse—his faithfulness had given her her sovereignty.

What is going on in those stories? Let's continue to read each of the characters as representative of a part of ourselves. In both stories, then, the main character might represent the conscious ego, while the frog and the hag take the role of the denied parts of the self—the parts of ourselves which we think are bad or evil, parts we don't want to know about, and try to hide. In both cases the "ego" or main characters have to be prepared to fully accept and merge with a creature peculiarly revolting to themselves. The ego is shown having to give up all its preconceived ideas, and let go of any notion of controlling its circumstances. But at the moment when it fully accepts the horror of its situation, the situation changes.

The stories exactly describe the process of entering a phase transition through letting go of an old belief. A young woman kisses a revolting frog, a young man embraces an ill-mannered old hag and accepts her forever as his wife. Neither could probably imagine a worse fate for themselves; and yet each enters consciously into such personal annihilation and the sacrifice of their cherished convictions, and self-descriptions. And we can do likewise, using the stories as illustrated guides, and trusting that something new will emerge.

PHASE TRANSITION AND TRANSFORMATION

Before embarking on the journey, we need to be prepared. First and foremost, there must be a problem which is otherwise unsolvable and as travelers we must be cognizant of this. We must also have the courage to seek a solution at all costs and the stamina to carry on to the end. If these preconditions are not met and accepted, the journey cannot be undertaken. If they are present, we can usually find the courage to enter the unknown and not look back.

Entering a phase transition is so frightening that it is only when we realize there is no alternative that we are willing to experience it. Despair signals the crisis point, the point of phase transition. As that point of utter desperation is reached, we surrender to our immediate experience and a transformation can occur. The essential feature of the moment of phase transition is its inherent emptiness. And the magic of the transformative potential is contained in the point of nothingness.

Any attempt to take thoughts, expectations, or desires with us into phase transition results in its failure. All conscious thoughts of how things could have been or might be in the future, all hope for anything better, any desire for another solution—all those thoughts interfere, fill the space, and destroy the magic. If Gawain had had the slightest hesitation in embracing the hag, the spell on her would not have been broken, and he would indeed have been condemned to live with her as a hag. His worst fears would have been realized. Similarly, the princess would have had to live with a slimy frog, instead of a prince.

PHASE TRANSITION AND MODERN SCIENCE

The new physics is no stranger to change and transformation. It tells us that neither matter nor energy are static, unchanging entities, but are dynamic, and constantly shifting shape and even description—from matter into energy and from energy into matter. In short, modern science tells us that transformation and change are fundamental to everything in the physical universe.

A phase transition occurs when matter changes its form; for example when water turns from a liquid into a gas upon boiling—a simple observable physical transformation which poses no threat to the observer. Light's "shift" from particles to waves is more subtle—and more threatening to the observer with an investment in a single, rigid description of the world—as it is in fact a subjective or perceptual shift. Clearly, light is light and its nature is whatever it is. We as observers of light, however, can perceive it in different ways. Turn-of-the-century scientists, faced with the undisputable fact that what is observed cannot be divorced from the observer, had to undergo a perceptual transformation themselves to accept the paradox they'd found at the heart of their profession. They did not undergo that change without a monumental struggle. The outcome was the passage through a phase transition which we know as science's shift from "Newtonian" descriptions of the world to the theory of relativity and "quantum" descriptions of the world.

What physicists discovered was that we have to choose how we are going to observe or measure. We can see either the wave form of light or the particle form, but not both at the same time. This discovery has implications far beyond light waves, extending over the entire "reality"—a dangerous word—in which we understand ourselves to exist. To accommodate the fact that we as observers choose what it is that we see, and that we cannot separate ourselves from our it, we must transform our own perspective and change ourselves.

Unfortunately, perceptual transformations are threatening to the ego because they demand subjective change. Nobody feels threatened by the transformation of water into steam—unless they are standing too close!—but it is quite otherwise when the demand for change is directed at our very personality. So while such a change does not actually threaten us physically as individuals in any way, the intellect has developed ways of perceiving the world which are deemed safe, and any change to that perception is viewed with great suspicion.

PHASE TRANSITION AND MEDICINE

Such a perceptual or attitudinal shift is, however, the cornerstone of the healing process. Physicians are intuitively aware that a state of mind exists in which healing is more likely to occur, but few will have personally experienced an attitudinal shift themselves. Doctors are as human as anybody else, and are therefore just as threatened by a process which would alter their understanding of the world. So there are not likely to be many physicians able to lead patients into the nothingness of a phase transition.

In the previous chapter, we talked about polar opposite attitudes in the context of the Cartesian world view and inferred a perspective opposite to the familiar biomedical notions. Ultimately, the shift in personal perception required for healing is identical to our earlier "inferred opposite," because it entails a shift from objectivity to subjectivity.

The healing perspective is a way of looking at the world around us. We will now try to define it more concretely in order to understand how the shift can open the door to healing.

All patients come to their physician with a problem which is ultimately generated by a distorted view of the world. Most physicians unconsciously collude with this perception, and try to find a solution which does not demand subjective change. Unfortunately, this approach often leaves patient and physician unable to tap into the healing process.

It is an astute physician who will help his or her patients see their problem in a more positive light. Where such a change can be achieved, any treatment which might be considered will be more effective. Unfortunately, few physicians have any idea how to encourage the change, although many have developed intuitive methods through years of experience. The following comparison (*fig. 1*) demonstrates the alternative mentality which must be adopted in order to initiate a healing experience. "Self" with a capital 'S' suggests the totality of an individual, consisting of body, mind and spirit, embedded in a social setting and a physical environment. "Self" is therefore infinitely larger than "self." The phase transition is represented by the gap between the two perspectives.

· CONVENTIONAL PERSPECTIVE	· PHASE TRANSITION	· HEALING PERSPECTIVE
· Illness has external cause (eg. bacteria or virus)	· phase transition ⟶	· Illness arises from "Self" (ie. no external cause)
· The doctor has the power to heal	· phase transition ⟶	· The power to heal lies within the patient
· The doctor has authority	· phase transition ⟶	· The patient is the only authority
· The patient is helpless	· phase transition ⟶	· The patient is responsible for changing

Fig. 1—Comparison of the different perspectives of illness and health, with illustration of the phase transition.

Part and parcel of the healing process is an integration of the healing perspective into our lives. In practice, it means that we must take full responsibility for our illness and abandon the often fruitless search for its cause. This change of outlook is particularly important today when the vast majority of stress-related illnesses have no specific external cause. The continuous search for cause results in never-ending expense and increased anxiety, adding to personal stress and worsening any condition. Furthermore, the whole idea that there is a "treatment" for illness in itself grows out of the assumption that patients are helpless—which disempowers the patient. *Any* form of treatment can therefore unwittingly block the healing process.

Unfortunately, our entire health care system is built on an assumption of helpless patients who need to be rescued by all-knowing doctors. As long as we as patients believe that someone or something is going to come along and fix us, we really have no incentive to take the leap ourselves. Radical shifts in attitude can only happen when we face the despair of an *un*treatable illness, and surrender to it. At that moment, the moment of surrender, a relaxation comes into the system which is experienced as healing, and we realize that we possessed the power to recover our health all along. We enter the phase transition in despair of our lives and emerge reborn.

THE CONSCIOUS PHASE TRANSITION

The major factor that keeps us from entering a phase transition is fear of the unknown. All our attempts to put off the inevitable are based on the simple truth that there are things we do not want to experience. The idea of annihilation is anathema to us all. Yet negative feelings, such as fear and despair, are quite as much a part of us as the positive feelings of joy and excitement. Ultimately, we cannot have the positive without being willing to embrace the negative as well.

While it is certainly possible to delay entering the phase transition right up to the moment of death, the penalty for doing so becomes increasingly severe. Whatever form they take, the delaying tactics may only serve to augment the discomfort we feel as we enter the transition itself. It makes so much more sense to give up avoidance and shift to a more creative view of the nature of our existence.

By allowing ourselves to move without resistance, we can enter the point of nothingness in a relaxed way and enjoy the experience for whatever it brings us. This idea is crucial when it comes to understanding the generation of chronic illness. Ideally we should be so flexible and relaxed that we never accumulate the stress that leads to disease. Truly relaxing in this way is a particular challenge because we are consumed by the fear of change. With this in mind, let's look again to our stories and see what they can teach us.

The stories tell us quite clearly that surrendering to change is a wonderful thing, that there is in fact nothing to fear, and that we should give ourselves fully to the experience of annihilation if that is what seems to be happening. In this way, mythology can work as a map to guide us through our personal terror. Sri Nisargadatta Maharaj notes the simplicity of the realm of nothingness when he says, "There is trouble only when you cling to something. When you hold onto nothing, no trouble arises. The relinquishing of the lesser is the gaining of the greater. Give up all and you gain all" (Sri Nisargadatta Maharaj, *I am That*).

An intellectual understanding of the process of transformation can give us the necessary courage to face our inevitable fear of change. With the map of mythology before us, we can walk boldly into the phase transition as a conscious act, and trust that we will come out the other side with a new acceptance of life. Our old mind-set will then be seen for what it is—one way of looking at things, not the only way.

Chapter Six

JACK

The pink spark

*J*ack came to us some time after being involved in a car accident. He was experiencing a lot of pain in his back and neck, was developing increasing numbness in his arms and legs, and was losing the use of his hands. Since his accident he had seen a number of different physicians and had undergone numerous tests. Despite unlimited access to all the technology of modern medicine, however, no one had been able to point to a specific structural abnormality which would explain his multiple symptoms.

Jack became increasingly frustrated as time went on and began to feel that he was floundering in a medical wasteland, abandoned by a system he believed was supposed to help him when he was unwell. Surely there must be a physician somewhere, or some particular investigation, which could identify the problem so that he could get on with his recovery.

The case illustrates the typical experience of the whiplash patient. In a car-centred society, few people get through life without an accident at one time or another. Unfortunately, the resulting injuries are often both devastating and undetectable by even the most sophisticated technology; victims are tested and tested until there are no more tests anyone can think of to do, and then they are tested again, consuming enormous amounts of healthcare resources for very little result.

Jack's case provides us a look at a typical example of a patient's journey through the medical establishment in search of a cure for their chronic pain. The first investigation following a whiplash injury is usually a cervical spine x-ray. People will often go directly to the hospital after an accident, even if they feel perfectly alright, just to have a doctor look them over. To provide reassurance, but equally for medico-legal reasons, and very often just to be seen to be doing something, the emergency room doctor will order an x-ray of the neck as part of his or her assessment.

In most cases the x-ray shows no sign of bony injury and patients are sent home, frequently with a cervical collar for comfort, and instructions to see their family doctor in the next day or two. At that time, the patient's physician will usually arrange a course of physiotherapy, massage, or possibly chiropractic treatments, not primarily out of a belief that such treatments will do much good, but, again, to do something tangible in order not to feel helpless—a behaviour pattern which can make the *patient* feel controlled and so become illness-promoting. And so the accident patient starts the long round of visits to various well-meaning professionals, none of whom may actually do very much to influence the disability significantly, while the very urgency with which treatments are asked for and applied may aggravate rather than cure.

Many patients intuitively realize this, but lack the self-assurance to leave the system alone and go home to rest—as animals in the wild will rest—until they are well. Instead, we are so under the sway of our belief in technology and so afraid to trust ourselves, that we seem instead to prefer to start a mad rush around to physicians looking for someone to make us feel better right away.

That merry-go-round of professionals is precisely the ride Jack went on. Over time, he underwent many investigations and procedures to no effect, and seemed to be getting worse in spite of physiotherapy, massage, and other treatments. On top of the unremitting pain and stiffness in his neck, Jack developed chronic tension headaches, so that it became more and more difficult for him to work. He found that if he stayed away from work his symptoms improved somewhat, but any attempt to work produced a marked exacerbation of pain. He began to get first worried, then frightened.

At the same time, his wife, who had at first been quite sympathetic, began to feel frustrated and resentful because he was not getting better and she was having to take responsibility for him, their affairs, their home and family alone. Predictably, she felt guilty about her anger, so that rather than sharing it she suppressed it.

Eventually, for the sake of further reassurance, not because he felt there was anything to be done, Jack's family doctor referred him to an orthopaedic surgeon. Jack had been coming in week after week, getting more and more frantic, and demanding some action. He felt it was his right to be repaired by the health-care system and could not accept the idea that no treatment could be offered; and of course, his insurance company was demanding some further validation of his continuing disability.

Under such circumstances, few family doctors can resist the pressure to refer, and the second round of investigations begins. Jack underwent repeat x-rays of the neck, x-rays of the rest of the spine and sacrum, and a C-T scan to rule out a disc protrusion in the neck. None of the tests showed any abnormalities, so Jack was returned to the care of his family doctor, reassured for the time being, and the appropriate letters were sent to the insurance company.

Some time later, however, he began to develop numbness and tingling in his arms and legs; he became clumsy and began to drop things, and from time to time his legs would buckle beneath him. Since these were new problems and suggested a pinched nerve, he was referred to a neurologist and the third round of investigations began. Nerve conduction studies gave equivocal readings—while there was clearly some nerve root pressure, there was nothing specific which would explain the symptoms, such as a discrete lesion in the spinal column, and so a myelogram was proposed.

Up to this point, the tests Jack had undergone had been at least reasonably safe; and none had any particularly nasty side-effects. X-rays may have long-term consequences, but for the most part there is no immediate negative effect. The myelogram was the first "invasive" and therefore potentially dangerous test to be ordered.

A myelogram requires that radio-opaque dye be injected into the spinal column, to show up nerve-root outlets and reveal disc protrusions or other structural lesions. The test is not without risk, however, as it involves inserting a needle very close to the spinal cord. It nearly always causes severe headaches for a day or two, and more serious complications can occur. Though doctors know that the diagnostic yield from myelograms in terms of operable lesions is low and so are reluctant to recommend them, in the face of pressure from patients somehow myelograms are frequently done.

SECONDARY GAIN

By now Jack's case had cost the public several thousand dollars in doctor's visits, investigations and treatments; and all to no avail. While he continued to believe that his illness had a specific cause, his doctor was becoming frustrated and others began to wonder if Jack was in as much pain as he said he was. Perhaps he was exaggerating his problems to gain sympathy, or maximize his disability benefits. After all, his circumstances before the accident were not ideal and Jack had every reason not to want to return to them.

Prior to the accident he had worked for the government in a job which entailed a good deal of heavy lifting and he was always straining his back or his knees. And because he had different interests, Jack didn't get on very well with his colleagues. In fact, Jack didn't particularly like going to work. In his heart, he had always wanted to do something else with his life, but felt trapped by his circumstances. He had a family to support and a mortgage to pay. As long as he was working, his wife could stay at home and look after their children, something which was important to both of them. Therefore any talk of Jack changing work arrangements, or retraining, was understood to be a taboo subject.

Looked at from the standpoint of his overall situation, then, Jack's accident was a god-send. He didn't have to go to work, and the insurance company looked after his financial responsibilities for as long as he was sick. If he were to get better, he would have to pick up his life where he'd left off. So while Jack naturally wanted to be free of pain, in fact getting well was not a viable option for him. This catch-22 situation is typical of many illnesses. In some it is more obvious than in others but the dilemma is often there.

To Jack's family, his doctor, and his insurance adjuster, his "secondary gain" grew more and more obvious, and he felt the insinuations of malingering were becoming obvious though unspoken—the more so because some part of him knew they were true. Nonetheless, he felt more and more angry as he felt their disbelief mount. It reminded him of something else. It seemed to him that all his life he had had to fight to be believed. As an orphan, brought up in a foster home, he'd found life difficult; and now, when it was really rough, the people around him doubted his integrity.

THE TRANSFORMATIONAL JOURNEY

Jack had an unsolvable problem. In some cases, the medical profession can prescribe a pill or a program of treatment which gets people out of such double-binds for a while—though in fact such measures only put off the day when the problem has to be tackled head on—but for Jack the profession had no answers. He had nowhere to go and life was not worth living as it was.

In desperation, and with no relief in sight, Jack became willing to consider throwing everything away, because he realized he had nothing to lose. He entered a week-long program at our centre and participated fully from the first day in spite of his initial skepticism because deep down he knew that he had to change or die. He jumped headlong into the phase transition with little in the way of expectations, and as a result experienced insights which fundamentally changed his view of life.

Jack started on the road to recovery with an attitudinal shift which can only be described as transformational. In the middle of his first session of acupuncture, he began to shake uncontrollably in the particular areas of his body— his arms and legs—which had been numb. This phenomenon, which we call "myoclonic shaking," is a common occurrence. It signals entrance to the point of phase transition and is one of three basic types of energy discharge. It is largely involuntary, and is often accompanied by a lessening of perceived pain (see Chapter 12).

The same shaking occurred in Jack's second session and continued unabated for the next twenty-four hours and into the third session, during which time Jack was acutely anxious and a little frightened. The shaking was accompanied by the release of powerful emotions, of which he had previously been unaware. He couldn't hold a knife and fork to eat, and spent a couple of very restless nights.

The third session was quite dramatic. He was already experiencing myoclonic jerking and shortly his breathing became uneven, and he began to rage and scream. We gave him a towel to wring, which he grabbed and twisted with frightening vehemence. After a while his shaking appeared to subside, and he held his hands up as if there were a ball between them, saying he could feel a tingling of energy passing through his fingers. All of a sudden, there was a crack like a small thunderbolt, and a pink spark leapt across the gap between his fingers, taking us all by surprise.

Later, Jack told us what he had felt. He saw himself "as a little boy trapped inside an egg-shaped casing," trying to get out by "banging on the sides of the casing with no result." He was frustrated, angry, and scared—it seemed that there was no way out. But then, "suddenly, with the passage of the spark, the egg cracked, and I was free."

Following the experience, Jack noticed that he was in less pain. He felt sensation returning to his hands and feet, and full mobility to his neck. These changes were almost instantaneous, and although he was by no means back to normal, the changes were dramatic and he began to look at the whole history of his pain in an entirely new way.

THE EFFECT OF THE ATTITUDINAL SHIFT

The power of a transformational experience can not be underestimated. Change comes from *within*, not from without, and the experience places the locus of control back within us, where we can recognize it as our own healing system being activated. Secondly, the experience can show us how we have produced our own illness, giving a direct understanding of the connection between mind, body, emotions, and disease. Thirdly, the experience stops the search for cause—illness which is healed from within must have been produced from within; there is no need to find a structural explanation. In one stroke, the notion of mind-body separation is eliminated and a whole new dimension opens up. We have all been brought up to believe that illnesses are physical or mental. Now this illusion is gone, and we can admit to the mental aspects of our physical illness without fear of being labelled neurotic. Finally, the experience frees us from dependence on professional help, thus paving the way for a useful life to be restructured.

The transformational experience is different for every individual and may be triggered by many different situations or therapies. For Jack, with the passage of a pink spark, the essence of transformation had taken place. But that was not the end of his story. He had, of course, much work to do to complete his recovery—physical rehabilitation, career retraining, and the healing of family divisions were the huge problems that would confront him when he went home. But with his mental blocks out of the way, he was ready for the effort necessary to make his life work. Two years later he finished retraining in a field he enjoyed, and he continues to be pain free.

Chapter Seven

JILL

The surgeon's nemesis

*J*ill came to us with severe headaches, neck, and arm pain. She'd undergone two operations and was contemplating a third if we could not help her. Jill had injured herself lifting a patient when she was working as an acute care nurse at a major hospital. As a staff member of a prestigious teaching institution she had every reason to believe that she would be given the best that medicine had to offer. However, after the customary conservative treatments—physiotherapy, traction, hydrotherapy, and massage—she was no better.

Jill then underwent extensive investigations including C-T scanning and myelograms and was diagnosed as having thoracic outlet syndrome, a condition in which the nerves going to the arm from the neck are thought to be compressed by the first rib and its surrounding muscles. This diagnosis prompted Jill's doctor to recommend the partial surgical removal of the offending rib, and she unfortunately consented in the hope that it would relieve her pain.

Jill's diagnosis and subsequent surgery offer a graphic example of the structural bias of mainstream medicine just as her later case history reveals the major limitation inherent in it. If medicine postulates a plausible structural cause, then its logic dictates a structural solution—but if there is an error in the diagnosis or causal assumption, that logic leads us to compound the error.

No doubt there was a structural abnormality in Jill's first rib, but conventional medicine's assumption that such an abnormality must be the cause of her illness overlooks the possibility that it might only be an *associated* factor—a *response* to injury and pain rather than its cause. In other words, such a "cause" is not cause at all, it is an effect. Jill had responded to her initial injury by tightening up the muscles in her neck and shoulder and that tension had led to the syndrome of nerve root pressure. So while her diagnosis—thoracic outlet syndrome—was technically correct, the treatment suggested to her confused cause and effect and denied the role of her own body in creating the situation, and its capacity to solve it. Instead, a surgeon took responsibility for a surgical cure. Taking what we've described as the "right-hand path," as the first son does in our myth, the surgeon in effect sacrifices his or her patient's body to "save" the rational diagnosis.

For Jill, the operation was a disaster; she soon became addicted to a number of pain-killing drugs. And though she and her surgeon might at that point have been forgiven for questioning the wisdom of surgical remedies for her pain, such questioning is rare in modern medicine. More commonly, patients suffering from chronic pain literally beg their doctors to intervene, to the point that these doctors may feel pressured into undertaking risky procedures of dubious value because they don't know what else to do.

That situation is a surgeon's nightmare. Though both medical research and their own experience may indicate strongly that surgical procedures in cases of chronic pain have a poor record, surgeons' basic structural training leads them into dangerous waters. In Jill's case, a second surgeon recommended the removal of the head of the rib. This section is normally left in place to maintain stability, but Jill's severe and continuing pain, appeared to leave no alternative to its removal. Once again the logic of the situation dictated further interference. When the assumptions of structural cause remain, then logic dictates further structural action. And so a second surgery was performed, this time with marginal improvement of the symptoms in her shoulder, though none in her chronic headaches. And the stage was still set for further trouble as the root problem of muscular tension had still not been addressed.

Not surprisingly, Jill developed a similar pain in her other shoulder. Again, such a development might have warned physicians that the problem was more than simply structural, but they continued to pursue the idea of a structural solution. Her next step was to consult a neurosurgeon. He suggested cervical sympathectomy, or division of the sympathetic nerves to the arm, as he thought she was developing causalgia, a syndrome in which these nerves become over-active. Though this diagnosis was probably also correct, Jill was now in a situation in which surgery had produced an effect seeming to require yet more surgery.

Fortunately, prior to this operation Jill was subjected to a test block with local anaesthetic to assess the possible result—which was a partial paralysis of her eye and no improvement in her pain. At that point, her physicians, wary of any more unsuccessful operations, asked that she go elsewhere for assessment and referred her to the Mayo Clinic.

The Mayo Clinic is an internationally renowned research centre in Rochester, Minnesota, where some of the best brains in the various fields of medicine assemble, and Jill had every reason to expect that if anyone could help her, they could. It is to the credit of Meridian that they realized there was nothing they could do, and told her that she should enroll in a chronic pain program.

When Jill came to see us at the clinic she was depressed, in constant pain, and addicted to various pain killers. She was also more than a little skeptical of alternative approaches. After all, if the best doctors in the world couldn't help, what could we do? However, she also knew that there was nowhere else to go and no easy way out. And that made her willing to do the hard work necessary to regain her health.

Although there are many different aspects to a transformational program, some of the most dramatic occur during body-work or acupuncture sessions. Buried feelings surface, and emotions and illness are experienced as linked. When feeling is so buried that memory is impaired, then the only message the body can relay to the mind is pain—and that pain can act as an invitation to the individual to face the pain and initiate her own healing process.

It was in this way that Jill began to uncover her feelings, many of which had been buried for years and years. Some were so painful that she had hidden them behind a mask of temporary amnesia. The only clue that the memories were there was the tension which pervaded her whole body, and which allowed her to cope from day to day. However, once she had decided to try to heal herself, acupuncture enabled her to release some of her tension and it wasn't long before she started to experience some regression to memories of previous emotional trauma.

During one fairly typical session, Jill felt her neck become extremely tight and found she could hardly breathe. The dramatic constriction was an exaggeration of a sensation familiar to her—the pain and tightness she suffered every day in the same area. The difference this time was only in intensity. Yet as the experience of throttling progressed, she suddenly let out a scream, realizing suddenly that she was re-experiencing being strangled by her first husband.

It was a horror which she had completely "forgotten," that is, long since buried under an armour of muscular tension. She later expressed absolute amazement that she had managed to blot the incident so completely out of her mind. With her scream came all kinds of related insights concerning the meaning of her neck pain, her feelings of suffocation, her hoarse voice, and her difficulty in expressing her needs. It was as if the feeling itself contained both the problem and the solution at once—re-experiencing the trauma immediately relieved the intensity of her pain; and she began to understand why she was ill.

In later sessions, in the throes of excruciating shoulder pain, Jill re-lived another significant memory. She recalled herself at four years old playing in a sandbox outside her family's home in the prairies, and her grandfather dragging her by her right shoulder some distance to a grain elevator, where he assaulted her. Her pain was again significantly relieved by the experience and her understanding of the connection between long-buried trauma and present physical pain underscored.

Jill began to comprehend that in fact her neck and shoulders had been tight for many years, but prior to her work-related incident, they had not been so tense that she could not get through the day. As long as nothing else went wrong, she was able to cope, but she was so tense that it was only a matter of time before something serious happened. Like Jack, she began to see that her illness was generated from within, and abandoned the fruitless search for a structural cause, committing her energies instead to the long process of healing herself.

THE DILEMMA OF STRUCTURAL DIAGNOSIS

It is important to reiterate here that while healing can occur through personal experience on the level of feeling, it does not necessarily negate structural diagnosis. When we first began to see such phenomena occurring, it was tempting to dismiss the structural model as at best misguided, and at worst disastrous. However, in time we began to see that we had simply stumbled across another dimension of who and what we are as human beings. The emotional model is no more right than the structural— they are just two different aspects of the same thing. It is not that the surgeons and specialists were wrong when they diagnosed Jill's problem as structural; it is just that structure is not the whole story.

In other words, the problem is not with the diagnosis but with the philosophy behind it. Objective diagnosis is the name of the medical game. Objective knowledge is the basis of our system of well-trained physicians and surgeons, and any hint of subjectivity is rigorously ruled out of order. But any individual who denies her own authority and submits blindly to professional intervention does so at her peril. There was something in Jill which was producing inner tension on a massive scale, and no amount of objective intervention—as she discovered to her cost—could help her. She was in a sense doomed to pain until she woke up to herself.

Chapter Eight

THE INJURED CHILD

Except ye be as little children,
ye cannot enter the kingdom

*W*hy did Jack and Jill get to a place in their lives where they were trapped? Why couldn't they change their behaviour, when the things they were doing clearly weren't working? How did they get stuck in such harmful patterns? We believe that the answer to such questions lies with an injured and frightened child inside us.

Peter Nunn was five years old when he lost his mother during the blitz in London. She was struck in the head by a piece of shrapnel from a bomb that exploded in their garden and was killed outright. But as a child Peter remembered crying for her only once. Though he knew she was dead, he felt nothing. He forgot the raid, and even forgot what his mother looked like. He felt in retrospect that his life seemed to start when he was six, and to all outward appearances he was unaffected by his loss. He trained as a surgeon, married, and began a family.

So what, one might ask, is the problem with denial if it works so well? At thirty-six, Peter found out when several things happened all at once to shake his world. He had begun to realize that his marriage was in trouble when the surgeon in a neighbouring town—physically fit but a very "type A" personality like Peter, and only a few years older—died suddenly of a heart attack. At the same time, Peter found himself crippled with both back pain so severe he often could not walk, and a constant pain in his stomach. Forced to rest for the first time in his life at such an emotionally grueling moment, Peter felt that if something did not change, he would die of the emptiness he felt in his heart.

Just about this time, chance led him to a book by Janov, called *The Primal Scream*, which takes the view that childhood injury is at the root of much neurosis and felt a deep chord sound within him. Soon, he found himself hobbling as best he could into the woods near his house where no one could hear. He tried to go back to that fateful night so many years ago and make himself feel what the five-year-old boy might have felt if he had been able to face his pain. The effort made him first tearful and self-pitying, then terribly angry, as though he stumbled into a bottomless pit of rage and frustration which had been building up in him all his life.

At the end of an hour or so, Peter returned to the house utterly exhausted with severe back pain and a pounding headache, but the tightness was gone from his stomach for the first time in as long as he could remember. He felt distinctly calmer. Peter's "walk" in the woods became a daily habit and subsequent forays produced similar experiences. More and more feelings came up, and with them snatches of memories of that terrible night, and finally of his mother. He could see her face and remember the house they lived in.

Over time, he realized that the tightness inside him was easing. People around him began to notice that he wasn't so uptight, so prickly, so easily frustrated. He started to care more about people, including his family. One day, after about six weeks, Peter went for his "walk," and nothing happened. He tried all the old triggers. He imagined the bomb going off, his mother being killed, but there was nothing—no tears, no anger—just a feeling of calm. He was ecstatic and thought that he was cured.

At this point, Peter had two blissful years. Then, as his old frustration began to return, he realized that releasing emotions and letting go of old tension patterns, while a huge step in itself, was not enough. The next step was to uncover the belief systems he had built up along with the denial.

In a child's world, punishment normally follows misbehaviour; and a young child trying to make sense of a bad situation will often assume that he has been bad. Otherwise, why would such a terrible thing have happened? Unfortunately, this explanation also gives rise to the belief that the world can't be trusted.

In Peter's later life, he felt angry at everybody. If things were going well he was alright, but if anything went wrong, he would fly into a rage. He wanted desperately to please people—and to punish them at the same time. Though for the most part, Peter was able to hide or control his destructive impulses, he ended up blaming the world for them. He wanted to care for people, but if they tried to come close he would push them away, determined never to feel the pain of abandonment again.

THE MECHANISM OF INJURY

Never to be hurt again is perhaps the deepest desire felt by the unconscious following traumas involving abandonment and helplessness. Closely allied is the curious instinct that tells us that if we feel happy, bad things will happen and we will suffer. Consciously, of course, we want to feel happy, but unconsciously we believe that if we allow it we will pay the price. Better to keep our distance than to suffer losing loved ones again.

The most dangerous time for people who have been deeply hurt as children and who have not worked through that hurt, is when things are going well. When we meet someone who genuinely cares for us, when our finances dramatically improve—when Fate smiles on us—our hidden belief systems often take over and make us do completely irrational things, inexplicably sabotaging our good fortune. After the first flush of happiness, we may feel strangely tight and anxious, as if all the old pain and anguish which we have denied wants to flood again into our consciousness. We want to, and often do, punish the very people who have made us happy, literally biting the hand that feeds us.

HELPLESSNESS AND ABILITY

Rollo May has developed a theory of childhood development which regards infants and growing children as caught in the contradiction between their natural helplessness and their natural ability. Theoretically, we begin life in a state of total helplessness and minimal ability, and move in our early lives towards maximum ability and minimal helplessness. All going well, this transition should take place quite naturally. May feels that adequate parenting consists first of protection and nurturing, and secondly of allowing the child to separate and explore the world as it is able. In other words, adequate parents have to perform a delicate balancing act between paradoxical responsibilities. They have to judge when to protect, when to rescue, and when to encourage independence.

However, using the intellect to assess the rights and wrongs of a particular stance at a particular moment can tie the mind up in knots. Logic and reason are often inadequate to a situation, so parents must be able to trust their feelings and intuition to guide them. If either or both parents have had to shut down their emotional natures, they may have no such guidance available. In such circumstances, they will usually fall back on the rules of their own upbringing, handed down from previous generations, and so perpetuate a rule-centred approach to bringing up their own children.

Unfortunately for all concerned, rules can seldom adequately answer real life situations, with the result that inappropriate decisions are made. Adherence to convention without the guiding balance of the heart leads to endless inconsistencies. Some of the inconsistencies have no consequence, but others can lead to disastrous results for the "helpless" child. Consider the following all-too-typical situations:

A father loves his son, but is unable to show him any physical affection, as he is uncomfortable with demonstrating his feelings and fearful of "spoiling" the child. The child *hears* that he is loved, but is not held or cuddled, and so *feels* unwanted, rejected, abandoned. Over time, he also learns that if such unhappy feelings are not suppressed, the little love which is shown may be withdrawn.

A mother loves her daughter but develops a relation with her based on her own terrible insecurity. Because of her own unmet needs, she cannot allow the child to explore and develop independently. If this anxious over-protection is defined by the mother as love, the child must either suffer guilt for rejecting it or suffocation and loss of self in accepting "love" thus defined.

A father loves his daughter, but has sustained a major loss with which he cannot cope—the loss of another child, a wife, or his health, perhaps. He tries to spare his child by hiding his grief, but naturally transmits it non-verbally nonetheless. The young girl intuits his unspoken feelings, but is unable to talk to him about it, or admit her own feelings. She thus learns that certain subjects are taboo. She may also realize that her father needs help, and try to look after him at the expense of her own needs.

A child is "abandoned" by a parent through death or divorce at an early age. Such a tragic bereavement brings the child face to face with his or her own helplessness. Unable to cope with such irredeemable loss, or the sense that he or she is to blame, the child pushes the pain down inside.

Such suffocation of feelings can lead to breathing illnesses such as asthma. If the child does not have the ability to meet the needs of the moment, it still has to survive, and does so by adopting a variety of coping mechanisms and belief systems to protect it. Each of these mechanisms is based on a denial of the pain of absolute helplessness. Let's consider the mechanism of denial for a moment.

DENIAL

When we are faced with an overwhelming situation—trauma, severe emotional stress, or the diagnosis of catastrophic illness—our natural response is to protect ourselves by denial. In such situations, denial is both useful and necessary as it has to do with our very survival. But denial can take many forms, ranging all the way from a stubborn refusal to accept the facts, to complete amnesia. And while some of these are helpful in the short term—at the level of an unconscious obscuring of the truth designed to help us cope—authorities like Shelley Taylor, author of *Positive Illusions,* draw definite distinctions between the positive illusions which contribute to a healthy psyche—and the repression which may inhibit growth and awareness in *un*healthy ways.

Denial protects us from that which we cannot bear to acknowledge; and any attempt to tamper with it can be immensely threatening. We may feel as though our psyche will disintegrate if we dare to do away with it. Denial can also allow us to avoid responsibility, to maintain a stance of "innocence" or non-involvement in the events around us. One of our clients, for example, came home one day to find his wife had left him, taking everything in the house with her, leaving him only a knife, a fork and a plate on the kitchen floor. Initially, the man stoutly denied that there was anything wrong with his marriage and tried to make himself out to be an innocent victim. During therapy, he gradually began to acknowledge his responsibility. As he felt able to face it, denial fell away, and he began to experience more and more of the pain—not only of his wife's abandonment, but of the abandonment he'd suffered in childhood. He was then able to see that his behaviour, which was largely motivated to prevent anyone from leaving him, had in fact driven his wife away.

TENSION PATTERNS

What are the physical processes that keep denial in place? How do we deny things? And what are the consequences? Wilhelm Reich was one of the first to show that feelings could be denied by freezing the body in tension patterns, which remain, trapping the body musculature and trapped by it, until the denied feelings are explored, re-experienced, and released. He called the tension patterns "body armouring," and developed a whole system of therapy (called Reichian Therapy) designed to release blocked energy.

Reichian theory forms the basis of most modern bodywork techniques. Think for a moment of the anxiety produced by having to stand up in front of others to speak. The heart pounds, the voice quivers, the legs tremble, we may even break out in a cold sweat. The "fear" so experienced can be conceptualized as energy, which can move downward to result in "knocking" knees, or upward to make the hair "stand on end." Likewise, the energy of anger may move upward and cause a stiff neck or a headache.

All these reactions are perfectly normal and are coincident with an adrenalin surge in the body as it prepares to face acute stress—the so-called "fight or flight" response. However, since neither fight nor flight is appropriate in most stressful situations, we will usually try to control the shaking caused by this excess energy surging through us. We will try to control our quaking legs by tightening various muscles. If this blocking becomes automatic and longstanding, the tension which builds up may result in chronic back pain or predispose us to back injury.

This defensive posture is very common. In fact, most people unconsciously lock their knees when they stand, and in doing so cut the vital flow of energy through their bodies. If you take a moment to stand up right now, you can check your posture for yourself. The chances are that you normally stand with your knees locked, with most of your weight on your heels. If you cannot push your knees farther back, they are considered "locked." Try unlocking them and bringing your weight forward so that the balls and heels of your feet support equal weight. If you feel any different—if you feel heavier, or your contact with the ground feels different, or you feel a flow of energy in your legs or your feet become warmer—go back to your original stance, and see how it alters the new sensations.

Reichian energetics and acupuncture energetics are closely related. Both systems work with body-tension patterns, which in turn are related to emotional make-up, personality, and belief systems (see Chapter 11).

BELIEF SYSTEMS

Feelings of abandonment might be totally overwhelming if it were not for the mechanism of denial. There is often no good reason why we should be abandoned when we are helpless, and yet we have to make sense of the situation somehow in order to keep living. We can choose one of two courses: either we accept that our parents are "bad"—an almost impossible choice for children to make, particularly given loving parents—or, we must make something up which allows us to see our parents as "good." To succeed in such self-deception, we must of course distort a good deal more than our immediate perception of reality. If something bad is happening, and we have to believe that our parents are good people, then it may seem that our only choice is to believe that we ourselves are bad—though children who are suffering may salvage some of their self-esteem and preserve their parents' "face" by deciding that the *world* is bad. Such solutions are the only real option open to us as small children, because we have no choice but to live with our parents and are dependent on them. If we are bad, or the world is bad, our difficulties are more acceptably explained.

Whichever explanation we choose, our trust in ourselves, in others, or in our environment is compromised. If the denial on which it is based is not challenged, this distortion will eventually solidify into a belief structure. For a lot of us the feeling of failure or inadequacy lingers long into adulthood, fueling our anxieties, running our lives, preventing us from reaching our full potential, and lying at the root of our illnesses. This distrust can later lead to hostility, suspicion and cynicism, a need to protect oneself at the expense of others and of the environment, believing "It's me against the world."

BEHAVIOUR PATTERNS—VICTIMS AND RESCUERS

Warped belief systems lead to the development of certain behaviour patterns. These behaviours allow us to maintain a sense of control of the world around us—to stop us, that is, from ever feeling again our original helplessness.

Neurotic behaviour patterns are well documented. In "Stage 2: Recovery" in his *Life Beyond Addiction*, Ernie Larsen describes human archetypes delightfully. He speaks of caretakers, people pleasers, martyrs, workaholics, perfectionists and tap dancers. The categories are almost self-explanatory. Caretakers look after everybody else. People pleasers would die rather than risk making anyone upset. Martyrs thrive on suffering. Workaholics can never relax. Perfectionists fear doing anything lest they fall short. Tap dancers never make a commitment. Most of us will recognize a personal archetype if we are willing to be honest.

Rather than digress into the various character types, which are well described elsewhere, we will discuss two polar opposites which we will call "victims" and "rescuers."

VICTIMS

In Pavlovian learning experiments, an animal learns to make a response at the sound of a bell—"learning" a completely arbitrary cause and effect relationship. Children exposed to a Pavlovian context learn that they have little or no control over events, but can only respond—such children see themselves as victims of circumstance.

"Victims" are people who have decided that they can do nothing for themselves. Their basic belief that they are bad people prevents them from achieving their full potential. They get stuck in the helplessness of their childhood, and their trust in the "good parent" keeps them looking for somebody to take care of them. Their natural helplessness as children becomes entrenched as learned helplessness.

Above all, victims look for a "miracle cure", telling everyone, "If only things were different then I would be OK." Paradoxically, however, they will accept very little real assistance. If someone starts to fill a supportive role, it won't be long before the victim sabotages the relationship—confirming themselves in their belief that either they are bad, or their helper is bad, or the world is bad so that they can go back to being victims again. Once victims are abandoned by their would-be rescuers, in other words, they can go back to being victims again and will therefore often oscillate between helplessness and aggression or abusive behaviour—between forcing "good parenting" and provoking the abandonment they fear.

RESCUERS

In Skinnerian learning, an animal presses a lever which produces a certain response, good or bad. A child exposed to Skinnerian learning learns not only that he or she has some control over life, but also that action is essential to make the world work. If there is a significant accumulation of denied pain, this idea may turn such a child into a "rescuer," or a workaholic.

Rescuers have decided that they can trust no one, and must therefore do everything for themselves. In order not to feel their own helplessness, moreover, they have to control everything around them lest the helplessness of others trigger their own hurt. Rescuers really have only these two choices: they can try to save everyone, or they can deny that others are suffering.

Physicians are educated rescuers who often devote their lives to rescuing the ill and denying their own pain. Unfortunately, the need to rescue or "fix" people can prevent them from admitting their helplessness in the face of untreatable illness—to the point of outright avoidance. Thus the difficulty many doctors have with chronically ill or dying patients. They may visit such a patient less often, or in extreme cases not at all, and will often avoid addressing the subject of death with them. Such behaviour amounts to professional denial, and is usually obvious to patients, who may begin to feel very angry. On some level they know they are being lied to, but since they are often in denial themselves, may not be quite sure what is happening. When both patient and physician are in denial, the physician's attitude may actively retard any possibility of healing, whereas experience has shown that when occasionally a physician does cry in front of a patient, a barrier is breached which can lead to healing for both.

Doctors cannot teach their patients something they don't themselves understand; and physician denial is more common than we might care to admit. Physicians cannot afford to confront their own helplessness as that would make them vulnerable to their feelings, and leave them feeling both useless and out of control.

Rescuers will often look for willing victims to care for and because they believe themselves bad, will often take considerable abuse from them. This situation—currently labelled "co-dependence,"—is often exhibited by alcoholics and their spouses, among many other kinds of relationships based on reciprocal role-playing. As long as the rescuer continues to "look after" and collude with the victim, such relationships affect a semblance of stability, for if the rescuer were to stop supporting the victim the pain in their relationship would surface and this is exactly the situation which the rescuer tries to avoid.

Depending on the destructiveness of the victim's behaviour, these co-dependent relationships can last for years. In fact, if neither rescuer nor victim ever challenges the mutual dependency on which the relationship is based, such a couple can be stable for life. Predictably, however, such relationships are vulnerable to either physical or emotional crises or the need of one or other partner to grow.

In such a cruel and complex interactive morass, chronic illness or physical pain can become the alternate power supply keeping the relationship co-dependent, but it can also be the crisis which forces the relationship to change. Both victims and rescuers are at risk—either may develop chronic illness, an illness which becomes a metaphor for their mutual emotional and psychic pain. And this pain or disease can, paradoxically, act as a healing agent to one or both partners and to their relationship.

CONSEQUENCES OF NEUROTIC BEHAVIOUR

Neurotic behaviours consume a lot of psychic energy. It is very tiring to have to be a workaholic, or a perfectionist, or a rescuer, and life does seem to constantly present situations which force us to fall back on our neuroses in order to stay in control.

Workaholics will tell you that they will typically work *beyond* the point of burn-out, using a variety of stimulants to keep themselves going until they drop. The interesting thing about these "coping" strategies is that while the particular behaviour is adopted in order to avoid the feeling of helplessness, the result of continuing the behaviour is likely to be illness, or *forced* "helplessness," and forced rest. The paradox is that *strategies designed to avoid something eventually produce exactly the thing they are trying to avoid.* But we all continue with these strategies because the denied injured child in us believes that this is the only way to be safe in a dangerous world.

We might conclude that the more we resist experiencing our totality, the more we are forced to experience the pain of our denial. One solution to the problem of neurotic behaviour is to become aware of the injured child within us so as to consciously make a different decision. Since helplessness and pain cannot be avoided, we could choose to experience them rather than have them thrust upon us in the form of illness. In that way we can be truly "whole." Paradoxically, when we consciously choose helplessness, and are willing to feel the pain of our childhood terror, the aloneness and abandonment, we discover freedom and the real meaning of "control." And so the injured child within, when re-discovered and embraced, can become the teacher and the leader of the adult.

Chapter Nine

OUR MYTHOLOGICAL PARENTS

Even the unwounded are wounded

*I*t would be a mistake to attribute all our childhood problems to bad parenting. After all, most parents do the very best they can with their children, and even so children may grow up wounded. In fact, it may be in the nature of parenting that childhood wounding occurs.

This is a difficult and contentious point, but the following myths may shed some light on the subject. These stories depict the shadow characteristics of mother and father archetypes. When we understand the truth of the descriptions, we are freed from the need to see our parents as perfect beings. And too, feeling the archetypes in our bodies, rather than analyzing them in our minds, may help us to recognize the shadow aspect of ourselves.

THE GREAT FATHER

Greek mythology is made up of tales of gods and goddesses, many of which have become beloved bedtime stories for children. This particular tale relates the origins of Zeus, the Great Father of Heaven and Earth, descendent of at least two earlier generations. In this story, Gaia, the Great Mother Earth, gives birth to Uranus, the Sky Father, her first off-spring; and Uranus lies with Gaia to produce many children. Among the children were three monsters, three Cyclops, and twelve Titans—six sons and six daughters.

Like many mortal fathers, Uranus felt threatened by his sons. He literally couldn't stand the sight of the first six and so threw them into a hole in the earth, hoping that would be the end of the matter. But Gaia, loving mother that she was, was so upset by her consort's behaviour that she gave the boys a sickle to kill him. Cronus, the youngest and bravest of them, led the attack. He cut off his father's genitals and threw the parts into the sea; then he released his brothers.

Thus Cronus established himself as the new Great Father, ruler of Heaven and Earth, and took his sister Rhea as his queen. As power corrupts and power achieved violently tends to reproduce its own violence, Cronus, like his father before him, was paranoid of rivals and imprisoned his brothers in the hole in the earth. Once again Gaia was extremely upset, but rather than interfere directly, bided her time while Rhea bore Cronus' children, waiting for the day when they would grow up and overthrow him of their own accord.

Not surprisingly, Cronus was aware of the possibility, and chose a rather novel solution, eating his children as they were born. As one by one Cronus devoured Hestia, Demeter, Hera, Hades, and Poseidon, poor Rhea became increasingly distraught. So when her sixth child, Zeus, was born, she decided to give the baby to Gaia to hide in a deep cavern on the island of Crete. When Cronos demanded to see his newborn son, Rhea gave him a rock wrapped in swaddling clothes, which he swallowed whole on the spot without suspecting he'd been fooled.

Zeus meanwhile grew up, and returned to his father's house disguised as a servant to effect his revenge. One day he gave the cantankerous old man a drink specially prepared to induce vomiting. After a few moments, Cronus ejected the rock he'd swallowed as Zeus, followed one by one by the other five children, alive and well.

This story clearly describes some of the more destructive aspects of the father archetype. The Great Father, represented first by Uranus then Cronus, is bent on destroying his own offspring. Zeus, on the other hand, turns out to have had some more acceptable qualities, though he was renowned for his quick temper.

The Great Father archetype can therefore be understood as evolving. First he stuffs his children back into the earth, as though back into the womb, symbolically disallowing their birth. At the next stage, he permits their birth but devours them before they can grow. Finally, Zeus allows his children to be born and to grow.

How many of us have had fathers who have behaved like Uranus or like Cronus? How many of us have "eaten" our own children for fear that they wouldn't conform to our expectations? How many of us have felt crushed or consumed by our fathers in one way or another? Mortal fathers not infrequently direct some form of antagonism toward their children, threatened by their youth and vigour.

On the level of individual consciousness, on the other hand, the myth of the Great Father can be likened to our denial of the unpleasant episodes of our childhood. The Great Father is the epitome of denial, hiding or swallowing experiences that threaten him until he is forced to vomit them back up.

THE GREAT MOTHER

Stories which clearly demonstrate the negative characteristics of the Mother image are not as common in our culture. The following tale comes from Africa.

There once was a boy who lived in a village in the jungle. Like most young boys, there came a time when he wanted to explore a larger world. So one day he plucked up courage and told his father, "I want to see the world." With his father's blessing, the boy left the village, taking only his dog for company, and travelled for several days until he came to the edge of a pure and pristine lake, right in the middle of nowhere.

The boy looked around and saw that there were no footprints going down to the water. Indeed, to all intents and purposes the lake appeared totally untouched. And yet he he had an uneasy feeling about it. He walked slowly around the lake, looking to see if anyone was about. Eventually, he found a huge house, hidden in the jungle nearby, but nobody appeared to be home. After a while, as he was quite thirsty, he gingerly scooped two handfuls of water from the lake, one sip for himself, and one for his dog.

He then climbed a nearby tree to wait and see what would happen. Soon the lad realized that his uneasiness was justified, for on the horizon he saw somebody coming, and as the figure got nearer he saw that it was a half-giantess. She lumbered slowly to the edge of the water and started to drink. Finally, when she had quaffed every last bit of the water in the lake, she began to wail and cry out, "I will never be able to slake my thirst. Someone has taken two sips of water from my lake."

After a very long while, the giantess stopped wailing, disappeared into her house and returned with a great pot, which she placed on top of a fire she had started in a nearby clearing. She began to cook an enormous stew in the pot, loading in bags of grain, rice, bushes, trees, and any animals she could find. Horses, cattle, sheep and pigs all went into her pot as the stew began to simmer.

While the great concoction was bubbling, the giantess went back into her house and the hungry lad saw his chance to have some dinner. He jumped down from his tree and clambered up another with a branch overhanging the stew-pot. From there he could lean down and reach the stew without being spotted.

Using his spear, he carefully withdrew a morsel of meat for himself and another one for his dog; then he waited. By and by, the half-giantess came out of the house, and sat down to eat. In a short space of time she had ingested the entire stew. But when she had finished she became very, very angry. She raged, swore and stamped around, saying that she would never be able to satisfy her hunger because two pieces of meat had been stolen from the stew.

The boy was terrified at the sight of her displeasure. Eventually her anger abated and she went back into her house and he quickly climbed back down his tree and ran home. On arriving back at his village, he found his father and told him, "I have seen the world".

In this second story, the Great Mother's dark side is exposed. She is depicted as having an insatiable and all-consuming appetite which leaves nothing for anyone else. We normally think of mothers as being selfless and loving creatures, and hold our own mothers in particular in this light even if their behaviour contradicts the image. Mythology however allows us to look at the negative aspect of the Mother archetype. It tells us that the nurturer has a very different side to her. The half-giantess, represents the shadow side of the creative and nurturing Mother archetype. This shadow side has a big appetite, which consumes everything in its path, and a wicked temper to boot. She is powerful, larger than life, and unpredictable.

The myths describe aspects of parental behaviour which are not generally recognized. Parents are normally considered unqualifiedly loving with their childrens' best interests at heart. At any rate, most of us normally wish to see our own parents in this light. If our parents didn't actually measure up, we probably rationalized or denied their imperfections rather than seeing them this way. The suggestion that parents harbour negative archetypal behaviours which are ultimately destructive to their children is, after all, a difficult idea, even in fiction. Its not that parents are deliberately abusive, although in some cases they may very well be, but that all children are inevitably wounded by the very fact of growing up.

It is the denial of this wounding which makes it so difficult for us to find healing as adults. To rationalize our parents' shortcomings, we tend as children to consider ourselves bad or unworthy. Such negative self-imaging stays with us, blocking spontaneous healing throughout our lives. The myths, however, tells us that this childhood wounding is *inevitable*—that some kind of psychological scarring is in the very nature of the parent-child relationship. With an understanding of the destructive traits of our parents (and/or of ourselves as parents), then, we can let go of unresolved feelings of hurt and anger which linger in our consciousness and move forward. Without it, we may be doomed to pursue lives full of unresolved conflicts.

Denied childhood wounds affect all our actions and are embedded in the structures we set up in society. Furthermore, unresolved traumas are passed on to our own children so that the crippling cycle keeps repeating itself, generation after generation. We are fortunate indeed if chronic or catastrophic illness intervenes in our lives, challenging us to transform our awareness and find our own wholeness.

Mythological stories can ease our passage through a period of crisis by pointing out the path for us to follow, and in this remarkable way, may become the medicine of the future. The healing process requires us to discover the dark side of ourselves, represented by the childhood wound, and to reintegrate these rejected aspects of our personalities. If we do not rise to that challenge we may remain ill for a long time.

MEDICINE AND THE LARGER PICTURE

One way to view the medical system is to see it as a surrogate for our parents. When things go wrong, the health-care system, as its name implies, is supposed to care for us. When we fall down and hurt ourselves as children, we can run to our parents for comfort. If we fall and break a leg later on, we can run to the medical system for treatment.

If we look at mythology again, this time putting the health-care system in the position of the Great Father and Great Mother, the first myth can be interpreted as cautioning us against modern medicine's dark side. Like Cronos or Uranus, its paternalistic assumptions can unwittingly destroy its patients' capacity to find their own healing.

Treatment often gets in the way of the natural healing response, blocking the transformative process the illness demands, and creating a dependency on medical remedies which is ultimately destructive. But the myth tells us that this is just a manifestation of the Father's personality—there is no way it could be any different. It is useful to remember this when it finally dawns on us that modern medicine, with all its wonderful technology, is a cruel paradox—care that "annihilates"—otherwise it is very easy to get lost in a frenzy of rage and disillusionment.

Yet though this is the situation, not many people are aware of it because, like the wounded child, we can't quite believe that medicine, which is supposed to be so very good, could at the same time be so very bad. It is good in that, like our parents, the physician helps us when we get hurt, but bad in that this helping hand doesn't really want to let us go, doesn't want to see us grow up.

In the introduction, we described a man with chest pain who received treatment from a doctor. This man was treated and reassured at great cost in time and money, but no one bothered to tackle his real problem, which was fear. Because modern medicine misinterpreted his symptoms, he ended no wiser than he'd begun. It's nobody's fault in particular that such an omission occurs, as nobody is aware of the problem of fear, which is common to both doctor and patient in most cases. And this lack of awareness is so endemic that the medical system cannot hope to account for the consequences of its own procedures. Unfortunately, we must suffer the consequences regardless. The destructive tendencies of the Great Father are with us whether we try to deny those tendencies or not.

In our second myth, the half-giantess represents the all-consuming aspect of the Great Mother. The myth tells us that it is in the nature of this aspect of the Mother archetype to consume the very being which another aspect of her is nurturing. The experience is not unknown to us. We all want to be loved and supported, but we fear the smothering which threatens to deny us our individual freedom. So while few of us genuinely fear being physically eaten or suffocated, many of us fear being psychologically devoured, or alternately left to starve, in a world of all-consuming appetites and impossible demands. For most of us, these fears we harbour control our behaviour and keep us locked in patterns which may themselves become "consuming."

If we were aware of the consuming nature of the great Mother, we could move beyond her control. Meanwhile, however, our medical system consumes more and more of our collective resources, leaving little energy or funds for anything else. We seem in fact to have given ourselves completely to the maternal voracity of the health-care system, hoping we will be coddled from the cradle to the grave.

ACTION WITH AWARENESS

Our medical system is very like a parent, in that it has the potential to damage us if we try to live with it without understanding its negative potential. Ironically, we only have a problem when we cannot or will not look at the whole picture and take responsibility for our own destiny. We need to grow up and be responsible for ourselves, but we live in the society of the eternal child. If we use the medical system when appropriate, and don't give up our personal integrity to it, there is no problem. But only by such independence can we avoid being swallowed by it.

Illness is a call to the transformative potential within us. We must proceed on our own path, guided by our own inner healer and refuse to give our personal power away to our physicians or anyone else. And in the final analysis, taking personal responsibility is all we can do, because the system is just the way it is, and because we are just the way we are. The institutions of our society mirror the cultural consciousness of the people who set them up, who are, of course, our very selves. Wounded, we have devised a system that reflects our collective woundedness. There is no sense in worrying about it, getting angry about it, or blaming ourselves for it. The paradox is that the system will only change when we stop trying to change it, and instead concentrate on our own healing.

By understanding the dark depths of human nature, and through awareness of childhood trauma, we have an opportunity to avoid the consequences of the dark side of modern medicine. When we clearly see that all our societal structures have a dark side, we glimpse the larger panorama of the culture in which we are enmeshed.

Chapter Ten

EXPERIENCE AND BELIEF

Experience forms belief, and belief forms experience

*T*here is another wrinkle to the problem of denial. It has to do with how experience forms belief and how we then deny our experience in order to bolster those beliefs. This is a vicious cycle in which experience forms belief, and then belief forms experience. In the grips of it, we quickly become unable to accept new ideas, concepts, and situations which conflict with our preciously held point of view.

Recognizing this mechanism has far-reaching implications. Every time we block aspects of our perception, denying what we in fact see to safeguard our beliefs, we have to tighten up. As Reich has pointed out, psychological rigidity necessitates physical rigidity, and physical rigidity necessitates an expenditure of energy which in turn depletes us of our strength and builds up tension, setting the stage for illness.

EXPERIENCE FORMS BELIEF

If we were asked, most of us would say that we believe what we believe because experience has taught us certain things about the way life is. For example, suppose we form an acquaintance with someone. Let us suppose—though actually such a circumstance must be admitted to be entirely hypothetical—that we have no prior knowledge of the person at all, and nothing about our new acquaintance triggers any of our existing biases. We might go into such a relationship with an open mind and heart.

However, as we get to know the individual, we will start to form expectations. If the person behaves in an untrustworthy manner, and this behaviour is repeated, we will

sooner or later learn to expect our friend to be untrustworthy. If we are treated badly over a period of time,
we may conclude that the person is "bad." Alternatively,
we may conclude that *we* are bad, and therefore deserving
of bad treatment. Or we may believe both. However we
explain it, our expectations will begin to alter our behaviour toward that person and will colour all our future interac-
tions.

BELIEF FORMS EXPERIENCE

In any future meeting, we will expect to be badly treated,
and will likely be a little less trusting and open ourselves,
alert lest we are deceived. After all, previous experience
has shown us that such caution is only sensible. Such
reserve is a natural defence. Later, seeming similarities
may lead us to "leap to conclusions," or judge a new situation as we've judged the old, before all the facts are in,
"slotting" our present experience with earlier ones. Or,
say our friend began to treat us well; how would we react?
We would likely either reject the overture out of hand, or
regard it with suspicion; and such responses would likely
elicit more negative behaviour from the other person. In other
words, if our belief about the individual is fixed and rigid, we
will continue to misread his or her behaviour, and reject their
friendly overtures, leading them to confirm our beliefs.

While it is certainly true that our beliefs are generated
by personal experience, that is only half the story. Once
we have a belief structure, it leads us to experience our
lives in a way which confirms it. For the most part, we are
totally unaware that all this is going on, and as time goes
on become convinced that our beliefs are correct, as we
notice that all our experiences tend to confirm them. Unless we realize that we have ourselves set up the whole
cycle, we develop unshakeable convictions.

RIGIDITY, STRESS AND ILLNESS

The well-known story of the oak and the willow is an
excellent example of the consequences of rigidity. The oak

tree is large and strong, rigid and unbending, the very epitome of solidity, and stability; its fellow the willow is just the opposite, infinitely flexible. When one day a hurricane passes through the area, the mighty oak snaps in two and dies, but the willow is able to bend in the wind and so survives undamaged. Likewise, the rigid personality appears strong and can keep going for years, but is in fact far more vulnerable to stress, and frequently suffers from those sorts of physical breakdown or disease which seem to defy rational treatment. To be flexible and "roll with the punches," we must be very conscious of the fact that our personal beliefs structure our experience, and must try to remain open to new experiences without judgement—a tall order. We have to risk being uncomfortable, making new choices, and trying new behaviour. How many of us are willing to do that?

THE SELF-PERPETUATING CIRCLE

Perception, feeling, judgement, and choice of behaviour are linked together in a self-perpetuating circle (*fig. 1*).

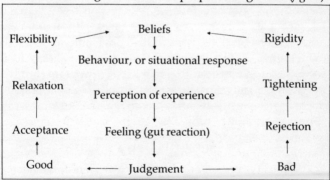

Fig. 1—Our experiences lead to beliefs which then structure experience—a self-perpetuating circle which keeps us in a psychological prison.

Our perception registers experience—which we must make sense of in order to survive—and that perception triggers feelings or "gut reactions." The mind looks to similar previous experiences and, if possible, categorizes the experience; then the intellect makes its judgement of it.

The category chosen has been previously structured, and memory tells us whether our experience is good or bad. At that point the gut reaction is judged to be one of two polar opposites—fear, for example, or excitement. It is well known that fear and excitement provoke similar physiological reactions in the body: both release adrenalin. So though our physical reaction may be much the same in two instances, the judgement made by our intellect may be quite different. If we judge the experience to be good, we interpret the feeling as excitement, while if we consider the experience bad, we interpret the feeling as fear.

This point is very important. A feeling is simply a feeling, but our intellectual interpretation of that feeling can differ completely from person to person, depending on their mind-set. As a result of our personal judgement, we make a choice about how we will respond. We actually have a choice of responses in most cases, although few of us ever exercise that choice. Our convictions colour our judgements, and define our actions as automatically as if we were a robot responding to a pre-set program. But the program can only run if the intellect presses the button— the intellect must categorize the experience before it can run an appropriate "program."

THE CONUNDRUM OF THE NEW EXPERIENCE

If we encounter an entirely new experience, we have a problem. The intellect cannot function without an appropriate classification and explanation for the experience. Krishnamurti once said that if we have an entirely new experience which the intellect cannot explain, then we have no experience at all ("Dialogues at Saanen," page 224 in *Talks and Dialogues*). Krishnamurti's statement points to a major problem. If our experience does not fit a category, we feel anxious. If we judge anxiety to be bad, we try to get rid of it by denying the experience. The effect of the denial is that —there appears to be no experience yet we are left trying to bury whatever feeling this "non-experience" engendered, and that effort creates tension and drains us of energy.

Chronic tension patterns are anxieties blocked before they come to consciousness; and the tighter we are, the less we are able to feel anything, and the more out of touch we are with our immediate experience. Eventually, we live entirely "from memory" as it were, governed by habitual beliefs and rationalizations. Any new experience is totally lost. No wonder our actions often don't fit present circumstances—our behaviour has become fixed.

Do we have to become ill before we can change this process? Another glance at our diagram will show that we can cut into the vicious cycle at any point, be it perception, judgement, or choice of behaviour.

CHANGING JUDGEMENT

If we judge a situation to be bad, we will resist the full experience of it by tightening up and trying to deny it. This is particularly true in the case of illness. The last thing we want to do is fully experience an illness; we'd much rather make it go away, and if we can't, we look around for a doctor who will. Fortunately or unfortunately, in the case of chronic illness, we eventually exhaust ourselves in the effort without achieving our end. We are left in a quandary. It seldom occurs to us that we could judge the experience of illness as *good*, because convention has taught us that illnesses are bad. So our dilemma is perpetuated by fixed belief.

If we could judge our illness as positive, however, a different outcome might ensue. A positive judgement would allow us to stop fighting the illness. To stop fighting it would allow us to relax. Relaxing will make us feel a little better, and that will allow us to begin to recover.

A remarkable paradox emerges: the moment we stop resisting the illness and experience it fully, we begin to recover. It seems so obvious on paper, but how many of us can manage such a reaction in the throes of disease? Not many! So we suffer needlessly, refusing to participate in our recovery. We remain in a disease-stricken mental state while waiting for a cure. Little do we realize that even if a physician could do something, it would likely prove a temporary measure, since the mental condition which leads to illness remains unaltered.

Wellness demands a transformation at the core of the intellect. Paradoxically, it is illness which often presents us with a wonderful opportunity to achieve this transformation. That sickness is bad is no more than an opinion—an opinion that leads to a particular outcome which confirms the validity of the opinion. If we consider it otherwise, we can experience it otherwise.

CHOICE OF BEHAVIOUR

Our behaviour indicates to the world who we are and what we believe. A doctor behaves like a doctor, and experiences the world as a doctor. It doesn't occur to her that she is just acting a part, because she really believes that she is the person she is pretending to be. What's more, she has persuaded the people around her to share in this personal psychosis.

When an individual who believes that she is a doctor manages to persuade everybody in society that she is a doctor, the whole society plays a part in confirming her belief. If we were to walk into an asylum, we might find people acting the part of KGB agents, or presidents, or anything else. These people are in confinement because they are the only people taking part in their psychosis. They have not persuaded sufficient numbers of others to share in their beliefs. Consequently, they are considered to have a mental problem and come into the care of physicians—who in fact are operating under their own invented identity, but who will probably never undertake to communicate with their patients by pretending to believe *their* psychoses.

One way to change our experience of the world is to dramatically change our behaviour in it. Achievement is often only the result of firm belief followed by continuous action in the pursuit of that belief. In other words, to become a doctor it helps to believe that one *is* a doctor, and to behave as such. Many accomplished people have adopted that improbable idea. That is not to suggest that everybody should start acting a part, but such transformation is possible at many levels—intervention at any point in the cycle can change our experience of the world. If we wish to change, we can. When we do, our experience of the world will change and with it, our beliefs. Neither we nor our convictions need be carved in stone.

Chapter Eleven

COMPLEMENTARY MEDICINE
SEEING THE WHOLE

The best medicine is no medicine

$\mathcal{W}$e in the West normally think of ourselves as separate, isolated individuals. So it's not surprising, then, that when we are ill we tend to separate ourselves from our illness, thinking of it as an alien presence, a thing in itself. It is "non-self," something to be *removed* from our otherwise healthy beings. This view is, however, limited and ultimately destructive. For underlying our perceived separateness from the things around us is a deeper connectedness. We are all embedded in a common world.

The recognition of this fact would profoundly alter all our present social structures, medicine only one among them. To change our philosophy of medicine and renew our vision of ourselves and the meaning of illness in this light, we must grapple with that connectedness, that common world and its implications.

SYSTEMS THEORY

The biological sciences have been brought into the modern era by what is known as "systems theory." In other words, systems theory has the same relationship to the biological sciences that quantum mechanics has to traditional physics.

Systems theory sees all organisms as systems made up of smaller systems, and considers those same organisms sub-units themselves of larger systems. The smallest system we might look at biologically is the mitochondria—the tiny particles which produce energy for cellular processes. These particles, which are thought to have once been independent living organisms have, over the millennia evolved a symbiotic relationship with our cells. They are nurtured by the body in return for their gift of energy.

The next unit "up" in terms of size might be the cell itself. A cell can be seen as a unit in its own right and as a sub-unit of a larger system. Cells of course make up our organs, which in turn constitute whole individuals. The interrelationship, at this level, of the part to the whole and the whole to the part is plain. To be healthy, a cell must balance its own needs and the needs of the individual, the larger "system," of which it is a part. If it does not, the larger system will suffer, and that suffering will in turn affect the cell itself. Ultimately, the well-being of the cell depends on the well-being of the larger organism.

Under normal circumstances, our cells effortlessly perform their functions in a way which is naturally harmonious with our overall good. Under certain circumstances, however, cells behave in a way which does not take into account the good of the whole. Cancer cells, from all reports, look very much like other cells. Their difference lies largely in their behaviour.

From one point of view, cancer cells might be said to be very successful. They consume the resources of the body with little concern for other cells, taking what they want, multiplying, transgressing organ boundaries at will, and spreading indiscriminately. In other words, cancer cells behave as though they have forgotten their integrated function in the whole organism. For the larger system, the individual, of course, such behaviour is a disaster; and eventually the damage to the whole organism backfires on these "selfish" cells.

THE GAIA THEORY

As humans we can be considered systems, and as such are sub-units of greater systems. The greater systems are families, societies, nations, races, humankind. As there is now much evidence to suggest that the earth in its entirety can be considered a living organism, ultimately we are sub-systems of the earth itself. The Gaia theory, named after the Greek goddess of the earth, embodies this idea.

It does not take a genius to understand that human-kind's behaviour is not suited to the well-being of the earth as an integral whole. In fact, homo sapiens might be said to have been behaving much like cancer cells for most of its recent history. It is perhaps significant that our cities viewed from the air look strikingly similar to malignant tumours seen under a microscope. Cancer cells' uncon-trolled growth is mimicked by rampant urban sprawl, and metastases by the "bedroom" communities surrounding large cities. As a culture, we seem to have forgotten that when we act against the good of the whole, we implicitly threaten ourselves. As cancer cells threaten the health of the individual, the individual threatens the "health" of the cancer cells.

Many people believe Gaia to be in the terminal phase of a cancer called "humanity." This being the case, from now on, her diseases must be considered a factor in our indi-vidual sicknesses. Given that there are very few illnesses which are not affected by stress, and given that chronic stress is endemic in our society, we must henceforward consider the influence of culture and environment a factor in every illness. Illnesses such as depression, anxiety, chronic pain, and cancer itself, must be understood to have cultural, ecological, and environmental contexts which go beyond the self. Yet what affects all members of a society is not likely to be noticed by any one of them—it is almost inevitable that we should ignore the evidence because we all suffer from the same blindness. And so a distortion is considered the norm.

Our cultural disease springs from our disregard for the larger system of which we are a part, and our medical system reflects our omission. Ultimately, we cannot solve our health problems until we resolve our misunderstand-ings; and because these misunderstandings are a problem

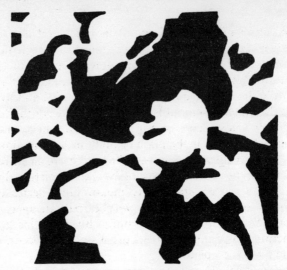

Figure 1

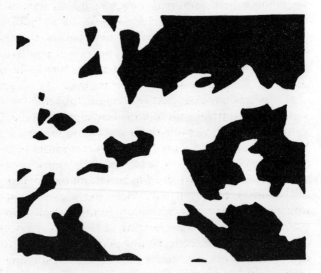

Figure 2

What do these random blobs represent? For the answer, turn the page.

(Reprinted, with permission, from Rupert Sheldrake's *A New Science of Life.*)

of consciousness, each one of us must find within ourselves the experience of integration into the greater system which is also a phenomenon of consciousness. A culture, after all, is made up of the individuals it contains. While the culture moulds the attitudes of the individual, so the individual moulds the characteristics of the culture.

How can we change our medicine to reflect a new vision? And what is the place of myth in the equation? Perhaps such questions can be addressed more easily by considering the problem of the blobs and the picture. Figures 1 and 2 are an apparently meaningless series of ink spots—unrelated, separate, without pattern, or connection. We see no picture, no unity. But if we stare at the picture long enough, a perceptual shift may occur, allowing us to see a picture.

A few people will see a design straight away. Some will see blobs at first, and then, in a moment of unfocussed attention, may notice a picture appear. Many more will stare at the blobs till doomsday and never see the image which is there, though once the picture is pointed out (readers who are becoming frustrated may turn to the next page) will rarely have any difficulty in seeing it ever after.

The experience of suddenly "seeing" the larger picture signals a perceptual shift or transformation. Imagine for a moment that we as individuals are a blob in such a picture. If most people cannot see the picture from outside, then clearly to see the whole picture—*while ourselves a blob in it*—must be acknowledged to be a monumental task.

The difficulty we all have in seeing ourselves in the universe explains our alienation from Gaia. It also explains our limited understanding of the consequences of choosing what we see to be our personal good above all else. Like cancer cells, we are in danger of destroying the body which supports us.

COMPLEMENTARY MEDICINE

Within our culture right now the concepts of "alternative" or "complementary" medicine are rapidly

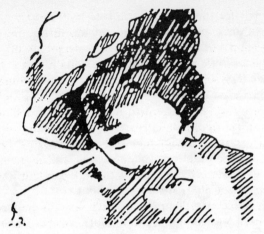

Figure 1 Answer

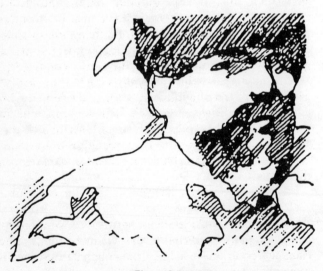

Figure 2 Answer

rising—for the most part outside traditional medical circles. Conventional medicine typically turns a blind eye to so-called "fringe medicine" and would ignore it completely but for the fact that it occasionally treads too close to its own well-protected turf. From time to time, for instance, the College of Physicians and Surgeons will see fit to prosecute an acupuncturist or two; and doctors maintain their traditionally poor communication with chiropractors and massage therapists. Naturopaths, herbalists, aromatherapists and iridologists as well as members of the general public are among the independent spirits who espouse the alternatives.

Whether such alternatives really are alternatives or just more of the same thing differently packaged can only be determined by examining each method and each practitioner independently. It is quite likely that many so-called alternatives are not very different philosophically from conventional medicine. Often it's a case of a different package, but the same contents. Furthermore, in spite of major differences, complementary medicine—an altogether alternative approach—is frequently confused with holistic medicine—which integrates the best principles of conventional and alternative medicines. Despite the bravado, the false revolutions and name-calling, however, there is no doubt that a genuinely alternative medicine *does* exist, and is here to stay, attracting more and more adherents as people discover the healing experience for themselves.

WHAT IS LIFE?

One fundamental difference between conventional and complementary medicine is the extent to which physicians will go to preserve life. Conventional physicians will often try to preserve life at all costs, citing the "sanctity of life," they feel is enshrined in the Hippocratic oath. Complementary medicine does not dispute the sanctity of life but asks, Which life are we talking about?—the individual self, or the larger Self of Gaia?

Most physicians are unaware that they operate from any belief system at all, considering themselves objective scientists. However, the idea that individual life is sacrosanct *is* a belief system—and one with specific consequences. Cartesian thinking sees the individual as separate from all else, and does not consider the connection between the individual and its environment. It is a view which sanctifies the individual, but disregards its integration in Gaia and the universe, favouring the individual to the detriment of the whole.

Such an imbalance, we are beginning to understand, must ultimately lead to disaster. The new systems thinking, notably, sees the individual as both separate from and connected to everything else—understanding that the individual is part of a larger system and the proper functioning of the larger system is every bit as important as the proper functioning of the individual.

The proper functioning of the larger system demands that the individual birth–death cycle not be tampered with too much as it constitutes the repair and renewal function of the next integral level "up" of the system. At the next system level "down," after all, the cells that make up our bodies are constantly dying off and being renewed. Stomach lining cells are replaced every three or four days; blood cells are replaced every ten to twelve days; skin cells are constantly being replenished; even our brain cells are renewed every seven years.

All this is an ordinary, seemingly unremarkable part of our lives. We are very little concerned at crushing to death millions of cells if we bruise ourselves; and even if at forty not a single atom of the physical self we knew at thirty remains with us, our sense of identity remains pretty much intact. We behave as though we were oblivious to the constant renewal within us, though if it did not occur we would not last very long.

The life of individual cells or smaller systems seems to us to be just not as important as the life of the individual or larger system. However, as cells relate to us as individuals, so we as individuals relate to the larger "body" of Gaia. Our birth and death cycles as human beings are part of maintaining the earth's vitality through renewal; and to interfere with this renewal is bound eventually to affect the health of Gaia, and ultimately, our own health.

Conventional medicine, which seeks above all to prolong the life of the individual has at its core, then, an imbalance which is extremely destructive to our planet. And we have reached the stage where the condition of the earth is critical. Without a fundamental understanding of and respect for the good of the whole, medicine is unwittingly becoming a scourge to the planet.

Obviously our underlying philosophy must be radically altered before it is too late. Yet our existing health care system supplies only numerous and ever more disastrous manifestations of this imbalance. Quite apart from the global threat of overpopulation, there are a number of problems which can be directly related:

1 / Increasing medical care costs; 2 /a growing elderly population with untreatable senility; 3 / increasing dependence on physicians and life-support technology; and 4 / the interference with the gene pool through treatment of otherwise fatal illnesses in the young.

When the problems of conventional medicine are clear for all to see, there can be no question that an alternate must strike a balance between respect for the individual and respect for the environment in which that individual is embedded. Elderly Inuit traditionally sacrificed themselves in times of hardship. When there was not enough food to go around, old people would walk off into the wilderness to die. Though unacceptable in most contemporary societies, perhaps, this custom honours an individual's relation to the good of the whole. What more meaningful death could there be than one which enhances the life of those left behind? Nowadays, however, many courageous individuals who want nothing more than a timely and dignified passing are thwarted in their desire by a society unable to handle death in any form in which euthanasia and suicide are punishable by law.

In a healthy body, cells do not seem to agonize over priorities, but give themselves to the life-death cycle spontaneously, without struggle. Only in disease states do cells begin to value their own lives over that of the whole organism. When disease and death were rampant, and our hold on life as a species precarious, our overriding will to live made good sense. But in today's overcrowded society, our passion to keep people alive at all cost is out of date. The pendulum has swung so far in favour of the individual—at a huge cost to our common environment—that we almost need an "affirmative action" campaign to redress the balance.

But redressing the balance between the good of the individual and the good of the whole is no small task. Our minds think, theorize, and problem-solve, but our best-laid plans always go awry, and every new strategy built on the old foundation seems to generate negative side-effects. In fact, we can be sure that our well meant "affirmative action" campaign favouring Gaia would run into trouble. The last forty years have seen many states strive to put the good of all ahead of the good of the individual and lived to rue the destruction of human freedom consequent on their laudable ideals. Balance just cannot be forced; in fact, the need for force signals that balance is lacking. Equilibrium must be achieved naturally, by the free choice of free individuals, if it is to last.

Given the impasse we are at, it is clear that many of the excesses of modern medicine simply cannot go on. No society has the financial resources to fund a system with no limits. We cannot provide new kidneys to everyone who wants one just because we can do it, without creating a society of medical and economical dependents. We cannot go on doing heart bypasses on everyone who wants one, when the balanced living habits which prevent heart disease are available to all. We cannot "buy" good health when we have not taken the trouble to look after ourselves. Nor should we expect society to provide nursing homes to keep physical vegetables alive for forever and a day—often against their express wishes.

The reader should not misinterpret these remarks. They are not meant to be cynical or heartless, but incontrovertible fact. Society simply cannot provide free services to save us all from ourselves, nor beyond a certain point to save us from our deaths. Countries which have tried to provide such complete care usually find themselves saddled with a public debt which eventually cannot be paid off.

CONVENTIONAL VS. COMPLEMENTARY MEDICINE

Complementary medicine must therefore take a different approach, somehow directing its primary attention to the needs of Gaia while at the same time understanding the needs of the individual. It must find and implement a new balance without the coercion which would result in totalitarianism. Alternative medicine must be chosen by patient and physician *because they know it is the best medicine.*

As what is best for Gaia is ultimately best for us, complementary medicine seeks to help us see the greater picture as part of the treatment for every problem we face. The perspective shift is both our treatment and our cure. When we recognize the reflection of the cultural illness which is in us, we already are practising complementary medicine. When we choose to explore our illness from a cultural perspective, we are already exercising the alternative approach. A greater awareness of our integrated nature is the key to healing.

Without this recognition and the direct experience of our interconnectedness on the emotional level, all cures are meaningless. The negative emotions of fear and anxiety which create the root energetic imbalances which lie beneath many illnesses are simply cultural imbalances manifesting locally in the individual. Complementary medicine must develop techniques to recognize the destructive potential of denied emotional experience and to address the imbalance by using the energy of these emotions directly.

TOM

Tom came to us after having had a quadruple bypass operation, so he was well qualified to comment on the experience of the traditional surgical approach to angina. In the open-heart bypass operation, veins taken from the patient's leg are implanted into the heart arteries, bypassing the blocked vessels, and restoring the blood supply to the heart. In his case however, the four grafted vessels in his heart blocked up again within months of the surgery, leaving him worse off than before. His disabling angina continued, but the surgery option was no longer there.

As a long-term workaholic with a bad smoking habit, who could not walk a block without getting chest pain, he had every reason to believe that his days were numbered. With his life clearly at stake, Tom finally made some hard choices which transformed his life. He gave up his job, quit smoking and drinking, went on low-fat diet and meditated every day. He investigated using herbs and vitamins to build up his immune system, began to examine his personality traits, to unravel the mystery of his childhood wounds, and began the process of inner change which leads to the healing experience.

Over a period of five years, Tom managed to discontinue all his medication, and now lives with little or no chest pain. He has little inclination to revert to his old ways, as he realizes that he would undoubtedly recreate his original disease. It was unfortunate that Tom had to have surgery before he realized that he could direct his own recovery, but few people will make the choice of self-healing until they have been through all the other options first. In that sense Tom, like the third son in the myth, had to face an impossible situation before he would risk transformation.

ENERGETICS

Numerous approaches have been used to enter emotional experience directly, but all share as their common denominator the principle of "energy" or "energetics." Energy is the word we use to describe how we feel. High energy feels good, low energy makes us feel tired. Energetic disciplines—such as body-work, bioenergetics, meditation, acupuncture, group therapy, gestalt therapy and craniosacral therapy, to name only a few—do not seek to explain our experience by laboratory tests, but accept feelings as valid and strive to connect us more deeply with our emotional experience.

The most fascinating thing about energetics' role in complementary medicine is that it involves no medicine at all. A patient does not go home with pills or potions or creams. Rather energy medicine uses a variety of techniques to allow the patient to pursue self-understanding; and while this process may initially entail a therapist or facilitator, it ultimately dispenses with any second party altogether.

What's more, complementary medicine is largely inaccessible to objective study. Whereas treatment is something done to a patient—a pill or a medicine or a procedure—healing occurs inside the self, entailing inner shifts which render treatment unnecessary but leave no outer mark. So, though treatment and healing are not necessarily incompatible but simply represent the opposite sides of our dollar bill, it is small wonder that many intelligent scientists question the validity of such approaches in which objective change is neither necessary nor desirable.

In short, complementary medicine facilitates inner change; and its experiential impact, when it occurs, amounts to healing, not treatment. Perhaps the aspect of complementary medicine most threatening to the medical establishment is the ability of those who have experienced inner healing to become healers in their own right. Needless to say, such people represent a palpable threat to the Aesculapian authority of the medical profession, and to everything the profession represents.

HOLISTIC MEDICINE

It is important to point out that while complementary medicine may appear "holistic," it is in fact only holistic relative to conventional medicine. It is not absolutely holistic. Alternate medicine is simply a complementary principle, a therapeutic strategy from the opposite side of the dollar bill.

True holistic medicine must take the final step—that of bringing conventional and alternative wisdom together in an integrated fashion. Holism is neither subjective or objective, and neither favours or rejects either. All medicine and all therapies—whether it be kidney transplants, energetic therapy, or anything else—must be part of it. It should be remembered though that while nothing can be "unholistic," a treatment which does not take a global perspective is likely to be disease-producing in the long term and this impact should be considered when assessing its usefulness.

Likewise, all existing technologies, procedures and treatments urgently need to be evaluated in the light of the needs of the whole earth. If a procedure such as open heart surgery were evaluated and found to be wanting, its use could be curtailed by disallowing public funding. This would not necessarily penalize patients; instead it might well help them to preserve their health. When being saved by surgery is no longer an option, the need for self-healing becomes apparent, leaving patients to face their illness and make the choice to transform or die.

Unlike Tom, these patients would not have the disadvantage of having had an unnecessary operation first, so that their transformation would cost considerably less in every sense. In addition, through the process of inner healing they might acquire the ability to go on and help others similarly afflicted. In this way, transformational change could rapidly build into a healing wave for our society and our planet.

Complementary medicine has no fanfare, makes little noise, and has no technological wonders associated with it. It requires little more than a sincere desire for health and a willingness to stop looking outside for a solution. It is cheap, ecologically sound, and has no side-effects. Such a simple approach to illness must surely have a place alongside the wonders of conventional medicine.

Chapter Twelve

ENERGETICS AND TRANSFORMATION

A curse is a blessing; a blessing is a curse

*T*he practical application of complementary medicine is through "energy," which is experienced in the body through feeling. Illness is an experience on the level of feeling, and it is in our feelings that we find its resolution. Transformation can begin to occur when we get out of our heads, and into the arena of *feeling*.

Conventional medicine, based largely on intellectual analysis, abstraction and generalization, can never grapple with direct experience, which lies in a different plane. When we choose to explore illness through energetics we go on a transformational journey in which our whole perspective on the nature and meaning of illness undergoes a profound shift. Unfortunately, few people in our society, whether physicians or not, have any idea what the energetic or "feeling" approach is, so in this chapter we will look at some of the techniques which people can use to gain access to their feelings. The following story is an illustration of the kind of transformation which can occur.

SIR GAWAIN AND THE GREEN KNIGHT

One day as the Knights of the Round Table were gathered together, a knight of formidable stature rode up, attired all in green. He roared a challenge inviting the bravest of them to come and chop off his head—provided that he might return the favour, so to speak, in exactly one year and a day. The knights were stunned at the stranger's proposal, and it fell to Gawain to uphold the honour of the Round Table.

The Green Knight dismounted, knelt down, and instructed Gawain to chop off his head. Gawain struck a mighty blow and severed the giant's neck; whereupon, to everyone's surprise, the collosal green torso bent down and picked up its head, which spoke this warning, "Don't forget your appointment, Sir Gawain. On New Year's Day, a year and a day from now, I'll await you at the Green Chapel." With that, he jumped on his horse and rode off.

Near the appointed time, Sir Gawain went dutifully in search of his executioner, and three days before the New Year came across a castle in the wilderness. He asked the lord of the castle where the Green Chapel might be. The man replied that it was just a short distance away, and offered the traveller his hospitality. Gawain was welcome to anything in his castle, he said, provided that in the evening the two knights would exchange everything each had acquired during the day. The young knight thanked him and readily agreed to his mysterious proviso.

Early the next day, however, after his host had left for his day's hunting, the mistress of the castle appeared in Gawain's bedchamber quite apparently intent on seducing him. The young fellow gallantly withstood the temptation, which his hostess did everything in her power to make irresistible, but in the end agreed to exchange just one kiss. That evening when the host returned laden with the game he had caught, Gawain in return gave him just one kiss.

The next day, while his host was hunting, the woman came again to his bedchamber, this time extracting two kisses from her guest, whose honour remained otherwise unblemished. And in the evening, the two men again exchanged their day's yield. On the third morning, however, the day before Gawain was due to die, his hostess came again to his chamber to waken him. She pleaded with Gawain to embrace her, and he as steadfastly refused, but accepted three kisses and a green silken garter for good luck. That evening, when his host returned, Gawain offered the three kisses but did not declare the garter. His host offered only a gamy fox in return, and questioned Gawain closely about the gifts he received.

That night they ate and drank till the wee hours of the morning. The following morning, New Year's Day, Sir Gawain made his way to his appointment at the Green Chapel, hearing as he approached the unmistakable sound of an axe being sharpened on stone. In the chapel, he was greeted by the Green Knight who, without further ado, asked him whether he was ready to accept his fate. Gawain readily assented and knelt down to receive the blow. The Green Knight lifted his axe, started the downstroke, and at the last moment stopped, complaining that flinching was not allowed.

Gawain readied himself a second time. Again the Green Knight raised his axe, started the downstroke and held back at the last moment saying that Gawain's neck was not in the right position. The taunting was more than Gawain could bear; he shouted to the Green Knight to hurry up and strike his blow. The Green Knight lifted his axe for the third time, this time completing the stroke. But the axe only nicked Gawain's neck so that a little blood ran onto the ground, whereupon Gawain jumped up ready to fight, saying that he had fulfilled his pledge.

But the Green Knight put down his axe, took off his helmet, and revealed himself as Gawain's host of the past three days, saying, "My dear friend Gawain, you are the bravest man ever to have graced this land. Put down your sword and let me explain. The first two blows were for the promises truly kept, the blow which drew blood, for your lapse the third day. I realize that you lied to defend the honour of my wife, and therefore I forgive you. You did not deserve to lose your life. Please keep her green garter as a token of this day."

The key to this story is transformation. To a medieval reader, the Green Knight's colour would unmistakeably signify his association with healing. Paradoxically, however, his frightening size and threatening demeanour represent the negative aspect of ourselves which we deny early in our lives. In childhood, we symbolically "axe" impulses we judge to be bad, as Gawain felt the honour of the Round Table depended on his chopping off the Green Knight's head. In doing so we enter, as he did, into an unconscious contract to deal with the Knight later in life.

If like Sir Gawain, we voluntarily keep our appointment with our denied self, we regain our wholeness. Most of us behave with less integrity than Gawain, however, and hope to avoid our appointment. Unfortunately, this is not possible. The contract is not one we can slip out of. The consequence of our defaulting is usually chronic illness— a disease which comes into our lives when we are least ready for it.

If we read the story carefully, we may notice something strange. The Green Knight's challenge seems a little crazy since he offers to have his head chopped off, while in the same breath announcing that he will survive the assault. Anyone could be forgiven for thinking that once his head was chopped off that would be the end of the matter, as the giant would be quite dead and unable to collect on his bargain. In the same way, we imagine that we can "kill" chronic illness. Conventional medicine plays the temptress, promising all kinds of treatments, including pain killers, tranquilizers, or surgery. Many of us will succumb to the temptation, hoping somehow to avoid or forget the appointment we have agreed to keep.

Our story tells us that each day Gawain received less and less harvest from the hunt, while having to accept more and more kisses. Similarly, we find that medication becomes less and less effective, while demanding more and more of us. Eventually we wind up with the equivalent of a smelly old fox. But the myth also suggests that it is possible to resist the seducer, and remain true to one's purpose. Most of us need help to behave in this way. Even Gawain was not perfect, but his integrity allowed him to go through his experience and come out nearly unscathed.

Perhaps the most striking thing about this story is transformation of the would-be executioner into a fast friend. Similarly, when we do our best to avoid the attractions of the easy way out, and maintain our personal integrity, our relationship to disease is transformed. We discover the meaning of the experience and learn that the threat of death, initially so terrifying, can turn out to be a wonderful friend.

It is this transformational experience that complementary medicine seeks to foster. Conventional medicine supports us only in trying to defeat illness, offering us the axe with which to chop off the head of the disease, so that we will have that year and a day before it strikes a return blow. Later, when we can no longer escape our appointment with death, it tries to sweeten our fate with tranquilizers and pain killers. Alternative medicine takes us on a different journey, towards a fully conscious appointment with our destiny and a willing acceptance of risk of annihilation and death.

ACUPUNCTURE AND ENERGETICS

It was when we first began to work with Traditional Chinese Medicine (TCM), acupuncture and body-work techniques, that we began to see phenomena we could not explain in terms of a rational or structural framework. We started by working with patients in chronic pain from whiplash injuries using the acupuncture points specified by TCM diagnostics. These points were very often in the hands and feet, far removed from the patients' back or neck pain. Occasionally, needles inserted in certain key points would bring overwhelmingly intense feeling in their wake, virtually forcing patients to express the content or impetus for that feeling. In addition to this emotional release, two other phenomena appeared: first, myoclonic shaking, and second, regression to early memories. The next section discusses how these phenomena can be understood in the context of energy or feeling.

EMOTIONAL RELEASE

Emotional release was the most common and perhaps the most comprehensible of the phenomena. Acupuncture seemed to facilitate the release of pent-up emotional charges as though the needles somehow bypassed the conscious or unconscious mechanisms with which we normally control our feelings. The expression of such deeply buried emotion can be a very scary thing for all concerned; and it will not occur without a great deal of trust and relaxation. Such an atmosphere is not typical of a doctor's office, but is clearly a key ingredient in the healing process. Patients who release their emotions almost always notice a marked diminution in their experience of pain following the release.

The expression of emotion can take almost any conceivable form, and the deeper the experience, the more the whole body is involved in its expression. A specific sound—crying, laughing, shouting, groaning, or virtually any other—will usually accompany a particular feeling, and give the therapist a clue to its nature. When we allow ourselves to lose control sufficiently to permit the expression of the "monster" within, it is not long before there is a perceptible change in our experience of illness. We begin to realize the connection between our inner state and the manifestation of our disease. This insight in turn engenders an attitudinal shift—spontaneous and unaided by the intellect—and provides a deeper understanding of the nature of the healing process.

Emotions are often judged as positive or negative. Joy, happiness, excitement, and compassion are considered positive emotions while anger, fear, resentment, anxiety, and guilt are considered negative. In our society, it is often inappropriate to express certain of the negative emotions;

and we have little choice but to suppress feelings we deem to be unacceptable.

Unfortunately, the energy required to suppress unwanted feelings has to go somewhere, and it usually goes into the body. Various forms of tightening or muscular tension result and eventually manifest themselves as pain or discomfort which we then seek to explain using structural diagnostic criteria. In TCM however, the phenomenon of pain is interpreted simply as an "energy block," a more accurate description of how the pain actually occurs. Conventional Western medicine was developed from the study of dead tissue. The idea of "life energy," or "Qi" as the Chinese call it (often written "Chi" before the advent of modern pinyin in 1979, and still pronounced *chi* by most Westerners), has no accepted counterpart. Our prevailing attitude is that if it can't be seen it can't be there. Without a conceptual framework which accepts energy at face value, conventional medicine seems doomed to total frustration in its encounter with the many problems currently linked to emotional stress—the problems commonly facing the average family physician.

MYOCLONIC SHAKING

The second phenomenon we encountered was myoclonic shaking, a coarse or fine vibration of the limbs, trunk, or neck. Myoclonic activity occurs in a significant proportion of acupuncture patients, especially those that are young and have high energy. The trembling is often associated with an emotional release, but it can as easily occur without any associated emotion. Physical vibration will often begin in an extremity—the hands or feet—and from there will progress to other parts of the body—the pelvis, trunk, and neck. When the body is vibrating, an astute observer can see which part is stiff or is being held rigid, and can then direct attention to that area. Occasionally, patients will enter a state of total vibration, in which the whole body is vibrating at once. When myoclonic shaking occurs it is a good sign—there is often a significant amelioration of symptoms following a shaking episode.

Once the trembling begins it can persist for some time, even after the acupuncture session has ended. Ceanne DeRohan (in *The Right Use of Will*) and others have dubbed the phenomenon "ignition" as it resembles a fire which once ignited continues to combust until all its fuel is gone. The conventional physician, confronted with such a phenomenon, might initiate investigations to rule out epilepsy, or be tempted to suppress the energetic discharge with drugs. We have seen numerous patients who have been given medication to control the movements which have been occurring spontaneously at home. Many patients who suffer from panic attacks, for example, experience spontaneous myoclonic activity frequently; if they are frightened by the movement, they may request that their physicians suppress it. Given that the phenomenon is a natural healing response, suppressing it only freezes the patient in a state of illness.

Myoclonic shaking is an experience which is both voluntary and involuntary at once, and might be defined as lying in the "no-man's land" between voluntary and involuntary action, at which paradoxical point also lies the entrance to the healing experience.

The intellect has numerous means of invisible control, and it is perfectly possible for patients to override the shaking intellectually, whether or not they are aware that they are doing so. It therefore requires some persistence and reassurance from a trusted facilitator to encourage myoclonic activity to occur. The facilitator takes the role of the Green Knight, encouraging the patient to submit to a potentially terrifying experience. Just as Sir Gawain has to lose his head, the patient has to lose intellectual control of the situation, remembering that when Gawain consciously and unconditionally submitted to his ordeal, he was paradoxically given back his life. Intellectual interference, however unconscious, defeats the exercise, and blocks the healing power of the experience. Ideally, the patient relaxes deeply and finds the inner state corresponding to the experience of effortless vibration. As it is actually only a relaxation response, many people find that given time and persistence, they can quite easily learn to achieve the state on their own. The barriers are no more than fear of the unknown, and the intellect's decision that such movement is not appropriate behaviour.

As spontaneous myoclonic shaking seemed linked to recovery from chronic pain, we began to use energetic techniques with other illnesses and over time noticed that a wide variety of illnesses improve when myoclonic shaking occurs, particularly when the trembling is associated with emotional release. Clearly we are witnessing the physical expression and release of blocked feeling—a significant "de-stressing" of the individual physiology—as though the illness is being literally shaken out of the system.

REGRESSION

The third phenomenon we encountered was regression, the re-experiencing of traumatic events. During acupuncture, some patients will experience visual or tactile images of previous events in their lives. The events, such as a car accident, are sometimes directly related to the injury, but can also be other events which do not seem relevant to the illness at hand, though the regression experience will often make the connection between a specific trauma and the present illness in a way which has a profound impact on the patient, giving insight into the meaning of their illness.

There are literally no words to describe how profound an experience that can be. Prior to such insight, illness has no meaning and is therefore resented. After such insight, the illness is more often viewed as a teacher and friend. The Green Knight changes from a fearsome character wielding total power, to a wonderful and generous friend. Again, in the healing or transformative process, the shift in perception occurs quite spontaneously, after which everything is different and yet nothing has changed.

Jane was suffering from a whiplash injury and was extremely frightened when she first came in for acupuncture. She had a history of depression for which she had received drug therapy, and a lot of pain in her arm which was not improving with standard treatment. As a trusting rapport developed between us, she gradually became aware of a deep-seated disturbance which she wanted to explore. In subsequent sessions, she re-experienced being raped by a trusted uncle. During the assault, her arm had been broken.

In regression, she noticed the sudden onset of arm pain, and realized that the assault was related to her current ill health. After this insight, her arm and neck pain completely disappeared, and her chronic depression lifted. Long-term treatment with anti-depressants had done little other than dissuade her from investigating her problem.

All three phenomena—emotional release, shaking, and regression—are clearly interrelated. They represent different forms of de-stressing which together serve to release what can only be described as "blocked feeling." Since ambient stress is the one cultural phenomenon which underlies virtually all disease, the experience of de-stressing can lead to improvement in almost any condition. Predictably, "blocked feeling" is none other than the "energy block" which in TCM is described as "stagnant Qi."

These concepts are extremely simple, yet have absolutely no expression in conventional medicine, which attempts to work its miracles with these doors to the healing experience all but closed, and chronically ill patients who search for healing in conventional corridors are usually disappointed. It became clear to us as practising physicians, that the significance of what we were seeing was staggering, so we set about looking for ways in which we could help each patient experience the same energetic phenomena.

Naturally, not everyone expresses emotion during acupuncture under normal circumstances, and not everyone is equally at ease in exploring the hidden reaches of feeling. Different people have different bodies, and different levels of intellectual control. If a technique could be found which would increase the percentage of people who experienced ignition, such a technique would pay great dividends.

We felt that the prime factor preventing the experience was intellect control, so we posited that if we could find a technique to shift the focus of the intellect temporarily, more people might break into a significant experience.

GUIDED HYPERVENTILATION

The technique we were looking for was readily at hand in the form of "guided hyperventilation." Most of us can remember hyperventilating during childhood games, and the dizziness which ensued. Children usually discontinue the breathing when the dizziness comes on, so that few have experienced the stage at which the intellect loses control. During guided hyperventilation, however, we want to get beyond the stage of dizziness, as our aim is to get the intellect temporarily out of the way—to shift the focus of awareness sufficiently to allow feeling to find expression. The process is best carried out under the watchful eye of an experienced facilitator.

Hyperventilation functions wonderfully to augment the effect of acupuncture, fogging the intellect adequately, while allowing patients sufficient autonomy to terminate the process at any time. Furthermore, its effects can be detailed in sequence so that the whole process can be described to the patient ahead of time.

A typical acupuncture or body-work session requires the best part of an hour, sometimes longer. Ideally, the patient should plan to have a couple of fairly quiet hours afterward as well. "Recovery" time allows patients to internalize their discoveries and re-establish intellectual control. The rational world of our everyday lives is far removed from the inner world of feeling, and we need some time to cross the bridge between them. In fact, the most effective way to explore the world of feeling is to immerse ourselves in it for several days at a time in the safety of a group of people all dedicated to the same purpose. This is not always possible, however, and we must fit therapy into our daily lives as best we can.

Obviously, the best results come from full participation in the process, as any reticence only blocks the process—when patients hold back, they get nicked by the Green Knight's axe. In order to establish the highest degree of trust and the fullest participation possible in the therapeutic relationship, a little time should be spent establishing rapport before a patient's first acupuncture session. The patient should be told exactly what to expect, and reassured that they are completely free to terminate the process at any time. Paradoxically, the intellect feels safe in relinquishing control when it believes itself in control.

Hyperventilation, or "breathing," can be difficult, as we must persevere through a short period of dizziness and discomfort. The process is begun by breathing deeply into the chest and abdomen at a good pace, exploring full inspiration and expiration, as if we were running a race or trying to recover our breath. Many of us have trouble with breathing fully, particularly if we are used to holding tension in our chest or abdomen. Emphasis on the in-breath rather than on the out-breath is usually more effective, although this is not an absolute rule. Emphasis on the out-breath can blow off too much carbon dioxide and will occasionally produce aching tetanic contractions of the fingers which can be unpleasant. In the end, the best breathing pattern is simply the one that works, and is most rhythmically comfortable for the individual.

Following consistent hyperventilation, the mind begins to get a little fuzzy, and there may be a slight feeling of nausea. That is the Green Knight's first "blow," which may leave us feeling that to proceed is not safe, at which point the intellect, fearing loss of control, demands that we stop. Here a facilitator can be a great support because some effort of the will is required and a few words of encouragement can make all the difference. We need to be reassured that everything is all right so that we can continue to the next stage.

If we successfully breathe through the first resistance, the next thing we may feel is a tingling in the fingers and toes. The fingers often become stiff, or immobile, particularly if the breathing technique has erred on the side of the out-breath. The experience of something moving through the digits is unmistakeable as though each were a garden hose with water running through it. This is our first experience of "energy" moving, and because it is so new, it can be missed entirely unless the facilitator points it out.

Within a few moments myoclonic activity may begin; the body will begin to shake in one place or another, trembling at first as a fine vibration in the fingers or toes, later developing a myriad of different expressions. This is the Green Knight's second blow. The shaking can be quite frightening and may increase the resistance against continuing. The tendency is to try to stop the experience by tightening up muscles or stopping full breathing.

While the fear of imminent annihilation is getting stronger each moment, the facilitator will encourage us to stay present for the third blow, and with sufficient trust, we may submit completely to the unknown. At this point loss of control is complete and all of a sudden, as if from out of nowhere, feelings begin to arise spontaneously from the bottomless well of our being. Breathing becomes sustainable without effort. We seem to move into an altered state of consciousness, a state in which emphasis is on present-time experience as opposed to reason.

Between the two states of consciousness lies a phase transition, which is experienced as a barrier we must pass through. That barrier is demolished by the Green Knight's third blow, and when he strikes it, we enter a new world. This is the moment of the phase transition, and the moment of "ignition," during which the release of blocked feeling begins to take place automatically, spontaneously, and with very little effort. Intellectual control has been voluntarily relinquished, and we begin to perceive our inner selves directly through mental, physical, and emotional expression. We exist entirely in the present moment, as the total expression of the feeling essence of ourselves.

In this state, the distinctions between opposites which have structured our psyche dissolve. Right and wrong, love and hate, joy and sadness, pleasure and pain all are experienced as different aspects of the same whole. Our need to distinguish disappears, and with it, we may experience a deep love for ourselves and those close to us. Our whole body feels new, refreshed, and fully relaxed. We feel togetherness and aloneness at the same time, and we realize the power contained in our helplessness. At a stroke, we have internalized paradox! With the passage of a few hours, the more familiar mind-set returns, with its recognition of distinctions and differences. However a subtle shift has occurred, an irrevocable change in our awareness. We know that at the root of everything, *all is one*.

Energy medicine forces us to deal with new concepts which contradict many of our cherished beliefs. That a doctor do nothing at all, that patients be their own physicians, or that the patient and disease are one, are ideas that at first glance may seem absurd; and yet in fact we must grapple with these paradoxical notions if we are to understand the nature of the healing experience and start healing ourselves. The far side of the dollar bill truly is the opposite of everything we know rationally, yet it exists. The truth is that healing implies wholeness, and wholeness implies the totality of perspectives. We cannot choose one perspective over another and expect it to work in all situations without introducing a distortion which eventually bounces back on us in unexpected ways. When we refuse to embrace all points of view, illness is the reverberation which brings us back to the truth.

Chapter Thirteen

THE PROBLEM OF TIME

There is plenty of time when there is no time

*W*hen we use energetic principles to reach the feeling response within ourselves directly, we find that healing occurs while we are in an altered state of consciousness, a state in which we are focused in the *present moment*. Past and future are somehow dissolved and exist with us in the present. Explanations are not only difficult but somehow redundant. The experience of healing speaks for itself.

Explanation is important however, because if the intellect can grasp its own limitations through rational analysis, it may become more open to altered modes of perception; and since altered perception is part and parcel of the healing experience, permission from the intellect can be a critical factor in allowing healing to occur.

The time paradox is a case in point. We live in a world of linear time in which the passage of time is measured by the clock. It divides our time, and therefore our experience, into past, present, and future, so that we conceive of our lives in terms of what we did yesterday and what we will do tomorrow. From the perspective of linear time, the present moment is an instant of no actual magnitude, like a point somewhere along the course of a line, it does not actually exist at all. Former students of geometry may remember this particular paradox from their school days— each point on a line though seeming "solid" is considered of *no size*, and therefore non-existent.

How can something that so obviously exists be defined in such a way as to negate its existence? Though no one can actually answer that objection, an astute teacher might point it out as an example of the paradoxical nature of the reality in which we live. And if it is difficult to challenge our perceptions of the self-contained world of geometry, it seems altogether too much to challenge time itself, in which we imagine we live our lives. We believe we live in linear time, in a world of yesterdays and tomorrows, although such a conception is no more than a collective agreement. We can use our principle of inferred opposites to suggest another, opposite, but equally valid perspective of time in which nothing exists but the present moment. If the present moment is all that exists, this thing of no size must contain everything in the universe, including the past and the future.

In his book *Space, Time, and Medicine,* Dr. Larry Dossey has written extensively on the subject of illness and its relation to time perception; and with a little imagination we can easily see how the linear manner in which we have trained our intellects to perceive time combined with the increasing accuracy of our time-measuring devices over the centuries can be linked to the accumulation of stress and the resulting stress-related illnesses which are now epidemic. Linear time is such an all-pervasive idea that we could be forgiven for thinking that time has always been viewed this way. However, we know that this is not the case. When clocks were first invented, the smallest measurable unit was probably an hour or so—meaning "now" might exist for at least that long. But the unit of time which our clocks can measure has become progressively smaller and smaller. Now we measure time in nanoseconds, squeezing "now" until it is a machine experience rather than a human one. As no one will ever measure nothing, the paradox of the quantifiable but technically non-existent present will remain, however, science is doing its very best—the nanosecond is so brief that it is measureable but inconceivable. It just is.

Technically, then, present time neither exists nor can be seen to exist. The trouble is that we can only function in present time and so must come to terms with the paradox that our lives are being run by clocks which currently contradict our personal experience rather than confirm it, and that we are attempting the impossible in trying to adapt ourselves to linear time. Our effort to do so has demanded that the intellect—that part of us which can comprehend the notions of past and future in which we choose to live—assume the role of master over our feelings; while feeling, which lives in the present, has no arena.

Consider how linear time rules every aspect of our lives. We get up at a certain time, rather than when we feel rested. We go to work at specified times, whether we are ready or not. We eat at specific times, rather than when we are hungry. We live by appointments, and get upset if people are late. We wear watches and glance at them frequently to make sure everything is "on" time, and if we get a little behind, we start to feel anxious.

Anxiety is the terrible feeling that tells us that there is something to be done but not enough time to do it, or that there are six things to be done and not enough time—yet many of us would feel quite lost if we had to function without a watch for a day. Anxiety about time generates time-saving behaviour and has spawned several generations of consumer items to help out; and so we *rush* out to buy ourselves washing machines, cars, telephones, fax machines, and computers, only to find that these devices have a way of increasing the time-pressure on us. The car which was supposed to free us instead traps us in endless traffic jams, so that people spend several hours a day just driving to work and back. Telephones intrude on us at all hours of the day and night, and computers have a way of doubling our work load.

We are born under time-pressure and we die under time-pressure, and the pressure is getting worse all the time. It is the most ubiquitous stress we know, and one which we are totally unprepared to deal with, often forgetting that—irony of ironies—linear time is a human invention.

Time, we must ceaselessly remind ourselves, *does not actually exist* other than as an idea, *our* idea. It has no meaning for any other life form on the planet; it was never a force in our evolution until the invention of the clock; and it is so foreign to our experience of the present moment that we must often block out the experience of life altogether in its favour, replacing it with a disconnected, anxiety-ridden, rushed, rushed, rushed kind of living hell in which we must hurry in order to catch up with yesterday, and so miss what is happening right now.

Worrying about the past and the future is virtually a definition of "anxiety," a disorder which is so prevalent in modern society that almost no one escapes untouched. Yet how many physicians understand the relation of anxiety to our unworkable cultural assumptions of time? Most are themselves too caught up in the rush! So a consultation with a physician for anxiety is likely to be disappointing. About the best a physician can do is to give us a tranquilizer to mask the problem, or suggest some time off work to get away from it.

We will do anything except look directly at the experience itself. Yet the truth is that the simplest solution to anxiety is to find a way to experience life *in the present moment*. That awareness is the foundation of the new medicine. In the present moment, feelings arise which allow the spontaneous release of pent-up emotional charges, a release which both transforms anxiety and brings insight into its root cause.

Given that the idea of linear time is a relatively recent phenomenon, and that our relationship to it has become stressful, it is interesting to examine one or two other perceptions of time from other places and cultures to see if we can integrate the various perspectives into a "holistic" understanding.

CYCLICAL TIME

Cyclical time relates to the natural rhythms of the world and of all the living things in it. For an individual, cyclical time reflects the biological rhythms we are all familiar with: eating, sleeping, waking, the menstrual cycle, and the cycle of birth, reproduction, and death, for example. In turn, these human rhythms are linked to those of the environment in which we live: day and night, the seasons, lunar and celestial cycles for instance. So-called primitive peoples ate, slept, and planted their crops in tune with such rhythms without the stress of following a clock. Cyclical time gave early peoples all the time they needed. They lived in the present, dealing with acute stress as it arose, and didn't worry about what was going to happen ten years hence, no doubt assuming that in ten years they would be doing very much the same things as they were doing in the present. Their world seldom experienced the rapid changes which today we take for granted.

Cyclical time can be described as a paradox in which there is changeless change, in which all events return to their starting point. For example, the cycle of the seasons—winter, spring, summer, and autumn—simply moves round and round, change occurring in the context of repetition. Without a need to change the basic routine of life, an individual simply adapts to the needs of the environment and becomes a part of the landscape. Many so-called "primitive" societies still live in that way today although these societies are being continually eroded. The indigenous populations of Australia and the Americas, for example, have a cultural heritage which connects them deeply with their environment. It is interesting to note that as we slowly awaken to our blindness and arrogance and to the destructive potential of our growth-oriented society, it is precisely these "primitive" societies which are showing us the way to heal ourselves. Dr. Allan Duncan, who worked as a doctor in the Yukon in the thirties, relates a story in *Medicine, Madams and Mounties*, about a white man and an Inuit which illustrates the point of differing conceptions of time. Every winter morning, the white man would shovel the snow off his walkway down to the road. It wasn't a very long walkway but each morning he got a good workout performing his chore. His Inuit friend watched with growing astonishment the man's behaviour. Eventually he commented, "You white men are crazy. All winter you shovel snow; wind blows it back again; soon comes the sun; snow melts. You crazy like hell."

Linear time never returns to the same place, since it is about moving forward from the past into the ever-receding future. Cycles and rhythms are acknowledged to a degree, but the operational directive of a life lived in linear time is toward change for the sake of progress, and without the balancing effect of a changeless background, this change has no anchor to give it a sense of purpose. The result is a society which is growing uncontrollably toward destruction. As we helplessly witness the degradation of the planet, we develop a sense of a past irretrievably lost to us. And indeed, living in linear time means that change is irrevocable, whereas societies which imagine time as cyclical do not experience "loss" in the same way. That is a difficult concept for us to grasp, because as a culture we cannot even imagine living in the present.

TIME AND THE DOLLAR BILL

Time conceived as linear is a construct of the intellect, or conscious mind. It is the mind which stores memories, and projects possibilities. But past and future *don't actually exist*. They are ideas only, whereas feeling is an experience in the present, where the intellect can never be. In that sense, feeling reads the "other side of the dollar bill," a perspective inaccessible to the intellect.

If the result of establishing linear time as our mode of living is that the intellect controls feeling, the reverse is also true—the result of living in the intellect and disregarding feeling is that we live in linear time. The paradox brings us back to the difficulty we encounter when using the new medicine to explore feeling, although in this case we have considered it from the slightly different aspect of linear time and the present moment. Again: before we can see the other side of the bill, we must first be willing to let go of "our" side. In order to experience the present moment, the intellect must voluntarily give up its control. We try to live without feeling, because life seems safer that way, but the penalty of that safety is that we have to store our unexpressed and denied feelings in our bodies as tension patterns. No wonder, then, that we feel nearly annihilated when we experience the full force of our emotional pain.

THE TIME PARADOX

A simple way of demonstrating paradoxical functions is to plot them on a graph so that one is represented at right angles to the other. In this way, linear and cyclical time can be structured as the horizontal and vertical axes of a graph (fig. 1), in which the two kinds of time exist as complementary. Graphing demonstrates our perception of duality where complementary aspects are mutually exclusive. Since linear time corresponds to intellect and cyclical time to feeling, our graph expresses the complementary relationships of both pairs. Just as past and future extend infinitely in both directions and contain everything, so the present moment extends infinitely and contains everything.

We can see from our graph that the present moment represents a point of no size along the axis of linear time. But the real education inherent in it concerns the more subtle point that the opposite proposition must also be true—*past and future represent a point of no size on the axis of feeling*. In other words, everything is contained in the present moment, including the experience of illness and the experience of healing. To understand that profoundly is to apprehend the essence of the healing experience.

Interestingly enough, the concept of a "present moment" description of disease syndromes forms the basis of Traditional Chinese Medicine, which describes polar opposites existing in the present moment as yin and yang (fig. 1). Yin and yang, like cause and effect, are complementary principles, but depict a completely different way of looking at reality. By representing them graphically, their relationship to the cause and effect principles can be easily grasped.

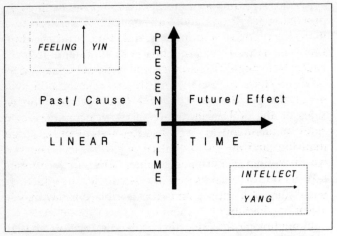

Fig. 1—A graphic representation of the complementary relationship of "linear time" and "present time." Past and future, cause and effect and "intellect" relate to the linear model, "feeling" relates to the present moment, while yin and yang encompass the whole.

Conventional medicine, with its emphasis on linear time, concerns itself only with cause and effect, a concept which fits our understanding of past and future. Modern medicine therefore has great difficulty comprehending the phenomenon of healing, which exists only in the present moment. We have mentioned that point before in a different context, and it is both fascinating and tragic that the same observation comes up again and again, no matter which way the picture is viewed.

MYTHOLOGICAL TIME

In order to view time holistically we need a concept which embraces both kinds of time and goes beyond them. It is impossible by definition to see both sides of the dollar bill at once, but it is possible to intuitively describe a larger reality that somehow encompasses both linear and cyclical dimensions. This brings us to a third kind of time—which is mythological.

Mythology stimulates the intellect and the feelings, by provoking intuitions about the nature of reality rather than describing it; and it transcends time, in that it both keeps us in the present, and takes us beyond time. Mythological time might therefore be said to lie in the gap, at the point of phase transition, and to reconcile the otherwise unsolvable paradox. It bridges the "void" between the two sides of the dollar bill, allowing us to experience both sides simultaneously. We describe mythology as larger than life, and as set in a place of "no time." The very words of the familiar opening line, "Once upon a time," take us out of ourselves to another reality in which the usual rules don't apply. In that magic place, a day may be a year or a lifetime.

In mythological stories, time is used to indicate change, transformation, or stages of development in such a way that linear time develops the experience of cyclical time; while characters represent aspects of our consciousness. A reference to the story of Sir Gawain will illustrate this difficult point. In the Green Knight story, Sir Gawain was given one year and a day to submit himself to his destiny. The statement seems to imply linear time, but clearly the "year" could represent any length of time at all. In any case, the story only deals with the last three days of that year, and focuses on the experience of the three temptations and the three blows. Why then, is the time *one year and a day* so important to the story?

The answer must be that something other than linear time is being indicated. From a mythological perspective, the year might represent something meaningful in cyclical rather than in linear time, and so bridge the gap between the two concepts. A year is the period of time it takes for the seasons to complete one whole cycle and return to their starting point. The reference to one year in the story then, reminds us that we too must return to our starting point in order to meet our appointment with destiny. The childhood wound initiates a journey into the sphere of the Green Knight, and we have to return to it in order to heal.

Significantly, the notion of returning to our childhood wound seems to be represented in linear time, whereas healing and transformation are linked to the flow of cyclical time. Mythology is like a collective dream where a lifetime can be compressed into seconds and a second can become a lifetime. We are all aware that in the dream state, time seems completely different, nearly non-existent in a way intellect cannot fully understand. What is very clear in a dream seems crazy when we wake up. Too often we dismiss the vital experience of another reality simply because it seems irrational.

Just as our individual dreams tell us who we are, and may point to our future growth, our mythological stories—or collective dream—tell us not only where we are, but where we need to go. Although modern psychiatry has attempted to fill the void left by the destruction of cyclical and mythological time, it is primarily intellectual and derived from conventional medicine, and therefore inherently locked into linear concepts of cause and effect. Thus it necessarily misses the "now,"—the moment of healing—choosing instead to attack mental illness with mind-altering drugs, which can sadly freeze patients in the middle of their healing journey.

It is hard to believe that something like linear time, which we take so much for granted and almost never question, could be at the root of our cultural imbalance. Yet such is the power of cultural conditioning that most of us exist as if in a trance. Even the scientists, who claim to be the seekers of truth, base their experiments on assumptions which are in essence insupportable. And we in our collective trance may only be woken by a massive upheaval which rocks the foundations of life on earth. And there is abundant evidence that this upheaval is in fact in the making, and that its result will be beneficial in the long run. Is mankind as a whole returning to meet its destiny at the hands of the Green Knight—or are we still trying to figure out how to avoid him?

Chapter Fourteen

HEALTH, ILLNESS AND RELATIVITY

To be good is to be bad; to be well is to be sick; to know
health is to know illness

*W*hen the paradox of healing is truly encountered, we confront a fundamental ethical quandary as old as humankind itself—*What is good and what is bad?* The question has defied rational solution for millennia but, fortunately for us, there was an old farmer who understood the problem very well.

One day all the old man's crops were destroyed by a storm. His many sympathetic neighbours came round to commiserate, saying what bad luck he was having. But the farmer simply replied, "Maybe yes, maybe no." Since he was running short of food without his crops, the farmer sent his son to town to buy some food. While the boy was in town he struck a good bargain and came home with a magnificent horse. The neighbours said how lucky he was to have acquired such a beautiful animal, but the farmer simply replied, "Maybe yes, maybe no." The next day while out riding, the son fell off his new horse and broke his leg. Once again the villagers commiserated with the farmer on his terrible luck. But the farmer maintained his composure saying only, "Maybe yes, maybe no." The next day the army came to pick up conscripts for the war, but because the farmer's son was injured, they allowed the lad to stay at home with his family. The villagers were astounded at the farmer's good fortune. But the farmer simply said, "Maybe yes, and maybe no. . . ."

The old farmer realized that nothing is absolutely good or absolutely bad, and both are relative to one another. What appears good from one perspective can often be viewed as bad from another, and because the old man knew this great secret, he did not judge his circumstances. More recently, another wise man called Einstein introduced the world to his theory of relativity. But despite the fact that modern physics has by and large embraced his ideas, as a society we have been slow to internalize them.

Many of us have fixed moral values based on our upbringing and/or religious beliefs which appear to answer the question of good and evil for us; and we often take those beliefs to be self-evident. Our governments, moreover, act as moral arbitrators, making and enforcing laws, and maintaining an elaborate judicial system to judge both the lawbreakers and the laws themselves. It seems fundamental to our culture to have rules and regulations of all kinds, and our job as individuals seems to be to get through life without transgressing too many of them.

However, as it becomes more and more difficult to devise laws which satisfy the sometimes conflicting moral values of different segments of the population, governments find themselves tied in knots and society is buried under an increasingly expensive and unworkable system. It is interesting to note however, that very few people question the need to have laws in principle—except perhaps in a case such as abortion. On the whole we still look to the law to solve our societal problems, whatever those problems may be.

Everyone has wonderful ideas about the laws they would make if they could, and politicians who gain power customarily waste no time in enacting their own principles as law, despite the fact that so often new laws only backfire, producing the very opposite of what was intended. And their critics in turn pose other laws which they say would be much better, without seeing that the same problems would result from any laws made.

Wise men and women, like the old farmer, know that they will never have all the information necessary to make an effective judgement about anything, so they usually refrain from making any judgements at all. And they know that since nothing is absolute, any hasty judgement will only prejudice them and cloud their vision, ensuring that bad circumstances remain bad as any opportunity to change them for the better will be missed. Similarly, illness and health can only be truly integrated by comprehending and embracing their relativity. The healing experience involves a massive shifting of our inner attitudes, which literally "turns us on our heads," and allows us to integrate conflicting perspectives.

As a society, however, we seem to be collectively blind to the limitations of rigid structures and totally unequipped to find real solutions. To understand this blindness, we must look to our childhood wound. Our need for rigidity and structure stems directly from our unwillingness to face the pain of our childhood experience. Mythology tells us that the wound is both necessary and inevitable—necessary to initiate the growth of the child into an adult, and inevitable to our individuation. Psychology tells us that it is passed from parent to child and is characterized by the inability to fully experience feeling, and a tendency to conceal pain by developing rigid structures, both in our bodies and in our society. It is a cross-cultural phenomenon which afflicts virtually all modern societies, and defies solution because—like the child—societies deny that the problem exists.

In denial, without the guidance of our feelings, we have no choice but to operate from our intellect—living our lives in the constant tension engendered by maintaining arbitrary distinctions, expending enormous amounts of energy rationalizing rules that conflict with what we know on a gut level to be right. Very often in our everyday life we must follow an absurd rule which does not fit the circumstances we encounter. Yet most of us choose to follow the rule anyway as we fear the consequences of following our heart—which can range from disapproval, to the loss of a job, or even death. In making this choice, we avoid the immediate consequences only to plunge ourselves unwittingly into another less obvious misfortune.

The continual subversion of our personal integrity results in chronic inner tension, draining us of vitality and leading to chronic fatigue and depression. And our rule-bound society tends to punish the very people who could help us. People who are closely connected to their emotional natures have the most difficulty contending with the stupidity of rigid thinking. They do their best to cope but find no acceptable outlet for their emotions. Sadly, pressure from society, friends and relatives may make such people seek "help" from the medical profession in order to "get rid of" these unwanted feelings. When the medical profession colludes with prevailing conventions which indicate that feelings are to be suppressed, the way is paved for a life of sanctioned drug-dependency. As a society we have judged people who are connected to their feelings to be ill, and judged those who are disconnected to be well. Thus a kind of inverted societal insanity is rationalized—and a greater tragedy than that would be hard to imagine.

The healing experience changes everything and changes it for all time. At the moment of transformation, multiple contradictory feelings which have been suppressed for a lifetime are present simultaneously and immediately accessible. Fear and excitement, love and hate, anger and compassion, all seem to co-exist in such a way that we suddenly recognize them as different aspects of the same whole, and abandon our need to distinguish between them. In an awesome expression of the paradox of relativity, illness—a threat to our life—forces us to face our life and make friends with our death. What was bad is seen to be good, and what was good, bad. At the centre-point of the transformation, we realize that illness is an ultimate good.

If illness can in fact be good, then perhaps our old value-system needs replacing by a new more flexible one—one in which the need for absolute judgement is transformed into a willingness to let the situation and the moment speak for themselves. A system of values based on circumstance rather than rigid prescription will allow us to judge an action appropriate in one circumstance but inappropriate in another. Thus the healing experience connects us to the still small voice inside us and awakens us to our personal and societal power and responsiblity.

RELAXATION AND TRANSFORMATION

Patients with chronic pain often discover that relaxation produces pain and increases tension, frequently causing them to stop therapy at the very point at which they might make a breakthrough. If the goal of patient and therapist is simply to eradicate pain through learning a relaxation technique, then the significance of this paradoxical pain can be missed. In fact, it is often a clue to the existence of deeper feeling, and a signal that a patient may be near the ignition point. Therefore, when discomfort occurs, we try to reassure patients and to encourage them to go forward "into" their pain, and through it into feeling and "present time."

It is as though the wall which represents the protective barrier surrounding the "inner self" must be breached; and there is no way of breaching a barrier which cannot be felt or seen. Most people with chronic illness have built up so many layers of defences and barriers—and then camouflaged these under further layers of protection—that it takes a great deal of patience, skill, and experience to negotiate the maze and reach the core of the personality. After all, if we had wanted someone to breach our defences, we would not have protected ourselves so mightily in the first place.

When patients first visit a doctor, they are usually looking for a treatment which will cure them but leave their defence systems intact. In short, they are asking the doctor to participate in their neurosis, a trap which most conventional physicians fall into very easily, since most share their patients' belief that illness is bad. Few patients realize the contradiction they face when they demand healing without committing themselves to achieving it. Patients who turn to alternative medicine are not usually prepared to face the challenge of real healing. When they find their defences threatened and their pain paradoxically increased as they turn to confront it, it can be difficult for them to persevere.

Though we occasionally see emotional release and myoclonic activity even in relaxation classes, without any other stimulus to those reactions, relaxation techniques really only come into their own after the transformational process, and not before. After the transformational experience, patients realize that they no longer need to maintain their body armour, though while protective tension has become obsolete, habitual tension may remain. Clearly, it is at that point that treatment programs in the form of relaxation can become truly effective.

ILLNESS AND RELATIVITY

Complementary medicine takes the position that illness is good, not because it is good in any absolute sense, but because if we are to break the power of the cultural trance, we must understand that truth is relative; and while we cannot make absolute judgements we *can* consider the consequences of holding one point of view or another. If we believe that illness is bad, we have no option but to engage in a power struggle with it. If our illness is a case of streptococcal infection, this conventional attitude, along with the conventional treatment, will work quite well. But if we are in chronic pain, and can find no specific cause, fighting it will simply lead to further muscular tension, which will perpetuate the pain.

In fact, because distinguishing good from bad is the root of much of our thinking, we are constantly engaged in such power struggles, and by living our lives in a state of constant tension, setting ourselves up to get ill. If, seen in this context, "We attract what we fear," as many people believe, we would do better to consider illness a good; and instead of struggling with it, allow it to take its course. Surely our energy is better used in the process of healing than in maintaining the disease matrix!

The paradox here, however, is that taking this course presupposes a prior transformational experience. Few people understand illness to be a good thing before they have experienced a crisis and have found the key to the healing experience. And if we know that illness is good, we are unlikely to get ill at all because, understanding that "There is nothing to fear in the universe" we will not generate the tension patterns which cause illness.

Everything in the universe plays its part in the whole; and whether we understand its function or not, we can be assured that it has its place. The old farmer understood this instinctively, but his wisdom probably fell on his neighbours' deaf ears. We will never look at the other point of view unless we have to.

Again, the transformational experience teaches us that illness and health are not altogether separate entities—an intuition with which modern science would heartily concur. The existence of one is entirely dependent on the existence of the other. Not only is it impossible to destroy half of our being, but if we were ever to succeed, we would at the same time destroy the other half. Destroying illness would destroy health, as we are slowly discovering in today's complex world. If we learn no more than that from our individual experience of illness, its place in the universe as a teaching agent can not be underestimated.

Chapter Fifteen

THE PROBLEMS OF PREVENTION

To prevent disease is to produce disease

*A*t the beginning of the story of *Sleeping Beauty*, we are told that a certain witch was not invited to the christening of an infant princess and that during the ceremony she stormed in and laid a curse on the baby—a curse which fated the child to die before her sixteenth birthday from a prick in the finger. Everyone apparently had stood stunned in the silence of the church until another fairy stepped forward. As it happened, she had yet to give her gift to the princess and promised instead of death a deep sleep which would last a hundred years, after which time the young woman would be awakened by a kiss.

The distraught king, a new father, determined to prevent the witch's curse from coming true by ordering that all sharp objects be removed from the palace. As we all know, however, he was unsuccessful. Just before her sixteenth birthday, the young princess found a small room in a little-used part of the castle where an old woman was spinning. As she had never seen anyone spinning before, she was intrigued and begged the old woman to show her how it was done. Very soon, of course, she pricked her finger on the sharp spindle and all the inhabitants of the castle fell into a deep sleep which was to last a hundred years.

The strange story of Sleeping Beauty's death-in-life sleep is probably one of the best-known fairy tales, but its deeper significance is rarely examined. The tale uses a simple story to illustrate a fundamental principle of life—that it is a fruitless or impossible task to try to prevent people from learning life's lessons, in other words, to save them from themselves. In this story, as in others we have read, the king can be seen to represent the prevailing cultural consciousness. As a father, he is so concerned at the possibility of losing his child that he tries to preclude all situations which might allow it—in other words, he tries to control life by force, using his intellect to think his way around the problem facing him. The young princess, on the other hand, might be said to represent the fantasy we all have about the innocence of life. As the father tries to protect his newborn child, society tries to protect its fantasy about life from any unpleasantness which might endanger it.

Our story, however, advises us that our attempts to protect our cherished ideas about life can only backfire in the long run—the king's very protectiveness of his daughter leaves the princess ignorant of life's dangers and paradoxically leads her to her fate. If growing up is a natural process involving both good and bad experiences, we must not be overly protected from the bad ones or our development will be stunted and we may pay an enormous price. The story can therefore be read to suggest that setbacks and disappointments are not inherently bad; and the prick of the needle which changes the princess's life for ever might be read as a stimulus initiating transformational change.

Western medicine's paternalistic attempt to prevent disease, and its interventionist practices aimed at eliminating it from a particular part of the body seek to protect people from life's lessons. Certainly, modern sanitation has proved effective in controlling such epidemics as plague and cholera and we have nearly eliminated smallpox, typhoid, polio and tetanus; and even hope to limit the spread of AIDS by promoting safe sex and clean needles. But when it comes to stress-related illnesses, in which cause and effect cannot be precisely demonstrated, we have a very different situation. Such diseases arise from the condition of the whole individual. Nevertheless, much of conventional medicine is directed at primary "prevention" of diseases in just this category, such as hypertension and cancer. It is here that the story of Sleeping Beauty, whose death sentence is parlayed into a kind of timeless sleep or suspended animation, can give us some insights.

We believe that prevention not only does not work, but is expensive and potentially harmful, dragging society into a quagmire of expensive medical testing to create the illusion of better health, which is at best only a kind of suspended animation. To challenge the authority of one of the world's most respected professions seems heresy, but to allow foolishness to pose as knowledge is worse and that is precisely what is occurring today. To illustrate that point, let's examine some noteworthy areas of preventative testing in common use.

CHOLESTEROL

It frequently seems that as new drugs and procedures become available, pharmaceutical companies look around for illnesses to help market them. If an illness isn't apparent, it is often invented, and funds are directed towards research which is likely to back up the need for the drugs. Scientists who produce results counter to the interests of the pharmaceutical companies risk having their funds cut off.

Hypercholesterolaemia is one of a new crop of such invented, symptomless diseases. As we have ways of measuring cholesterol, and drugs to lower it, treatment of hypercholesterolaemia is now the norm. The real story, however, is more complicated than such practices might indicate.

It has been demonstrated conclusively that people with high cholesterol have a higher risk of cardio-vascular disease. Conversely, a low cholesterol seems to have a cardio-protective effect. Logic tells us that lowering certain people's cholesterol levels through diet or drugs would be a good thing to do. It ought to put them in a lower risk category. But does it? Although there has been more money poured into hypercholesterolaemia research than almost any other in the history of conventional medicine, the results have been far from convincing in terms of favouring any drug treatment. At least two major cholesterol studies of the past few years have clearly demonstrated that intervention produces no overall change in mortality rate.

The Lipid Research Clinics Coronary Trial and the Helsinki Heart Study both demonstrated a significant reduction in coronary heart disease mortality (19% and 34% respectively) over fifteen years, but reported sufficient *other* deaths—by accident and suicide—in the treatment groups to more than make up the difference. In other words, mortality went up a little in the treatment groups. Even if there were no biological explanation for such an increase in deaths, seen holistically, the fact that the overall mortality was not decreased is a major concern.

Although the cholesterol myth has been thoroughly exposed in the mainstream media, the unquestioned cycle of diagnosis and treatment goes on. In 1989, *The Atlantic Monthly* published a well-researched article by Thomas Moore, entitled "The Cholesterol Myth". Such findings have done little to change the treatment which physicians advocate for people with high cholesterol—no matter what the benefit, and no matter what the cost. As disturbing as any other revelation in Moore's article was the cost-benefit analysis of cholesterol screening, something most researchers ignore. His calculations make it clear that even if treatment were effective—which is questionable—the cost of forestalling one heart attack was in the region of $650,000. And yet, the medical establishment still recommends cholesterol screening and dietary control, and failing that, drug treatment, because our "logical" scientific minds won't accept the ambiguous results.

Meanwhile the evidence is mounting that while the commonly recommended diet-and-drugs regimen has very little effect on patients, transformative personal change *can* reduce cholesterol, decrease angina symptoms, and reverse atherosclerotic disease. Data from the "Lifestyle Heart Trial" run by Dr. Dean Ornish suggests that profound changes in patients' lifestyle and attitude and not piecemeal bodily ones are necessary to reverse heart disease, and that standard treatment regimens in the absence of these are comparatively ineffectual. Not surprisingly, physicians find it easier to follow the commonly accepted recommendations, believing that sweeping personal transformation in the general population is an unrealistic goal.

HYPERTENSION

Diagnosing and treating hypertension has always been justified as effective prevention of long-term complications such as heart attack, stroke and kidney failure. Yet while it is true that treatment appears to reduce the incidence of strokes, there is little evidence that it does much to prevent heart attacks, while producing side-effects which can make the treatment worse than the disease. In fact, moderate hypertension does not make the individual feel unwell and therefore cannot actually be called a disease at all. There is little evidence in favour of treating mild to moderate cases; and interestingly, hypertension in the elderly may even have a slight *protective* effect.

It is, again, a largely invented affliction, which the medical profession discovered when it started measuring blood pressure; and which pharmaceutical companies were glad to promote through intensive advertising and through funding research which suggested a benefit from drugs capable of reducing it. The medical profession rejoiced in the discovery of a relatively simple model of an "illness" which it could treat effectively, offering often frustrated modern physicians a chance to satisfy their eternal desire to be useful. With so much to gain, it is not surprising that treatment of hypertension has become the norm, albeit on flimsy grounds.

The truth is, however, that nobody comes to the doctor complaining of their blood pressure; they come feeling ill. The problem which lies behind hypertension is almost always an inner anxiety which the doctor colludes with the patient in denying. More often than not, patients go away with a diagnosis of hypertension and drugs to treat it, while the question of feeling ill remains and is sometimes even exacerbated. Some of the drugs used for years in this mock battle (diuretics, for example) have actually been shown to harm health in the long term. Instead of questioning whether hypertension need be treated at all, however, we have merely switched to different drugs, whose long-term side-effects are unknown. Better the devil we *don't* know than the one we do, it seems. Many of the newer drugs are known to have deleterious effects in the short-term, raising cholesterol levels, aggravating peripheral vascular disease, interfering with glucose metabolism, causing impotence, and even ironically, increasing the heart attack rate; but in spite of it all, doctors continue to prescribe them.[1]

The cost-benefit analysis here is also problematic, especially combined with such health risks. It has been shown that even where treatment seems to offer some concrete benefit—for instance in reducing the incidence of strokes—the amount of drug therapy required before there is any significant effect is enormous. The British Medical Research Council trial in mild hypertension showed that 850 patient-years of antihypertensive therapy were required to prevent one stroke.

MAMMOGRAMS

Several early studies of screening mammography showed reduced breast cancer mortality in women over the age of fifty. As a result, it is now widely recommended that women over fifty are screened annually, and in fact, many doctors recommend annual screening after forty. If mammograms can identify a breast cancer when it is too small to be felt, it seems only logical to assume that intensive screening will mean more early treatment and improved survival.

However the issue is not quite so simple. After the fanfare of those earlier studies, scant attention has been paid to subsequent trials which fail to show significant benefit in any age group. Ironically, some of the later studies have actually shown increased mortality in treatment groups. For instance, the Malmo Screening Trial in Sweden, involving tens of thousands of women, showed a higher mortality from breast cancer in women under fifty-five who were screened by mammography than those who weren't. And this disturbing finding was confirmed by the more recent Canadian National Breast Screening Study. But instead of questioning the wisdom of mass screening, researchers try to explain the findings of these studies away; many doctors continue to recommend annual screening; and unfortunately, patients just do as they are told.

Perhaps more to the point, is that even the impressive 30% fall in breast cancer mortality often quoted to justify screening is really much ado about nothing, because the figures are relative. *The Lancet* quotes the following example: if 10,000 women are screened, 1500 (10-15%) might have a positive screen. Of those, 137 (1.37%) will be found to have cancer. Of those, if eleven die in the treatment group, and 15 die in the control group, then it is generally interpreted as an approximate 30% drop in mortality. In reality, it is a minuscule 0.04% drop, since only four women have benefitted out of the original 10,000 screened. Looked at in this way, and averaging the results of several trials, it works out that 20,000 mammograms must be performed at a cost of $1.2 million, for each life presumed saved; and this conclusion still ignores the fact that, in all those trials the overall mortality didn't change one iota.[2]

It is natural to want to find something to help the scourge of breast cancer, and no one argues about the benefits of mammography as a diagnostic tool, but screening healthy people is not the answer. The worst of it is that mammography is not necessarily harmless. It beams radiation—which in itself can cause cancer—into the breasts, and requires breast compression, which may contribute to the spread of any pre-existing cancer cells.[3] It can be painful, is anxiety-provoking, produces false negatives—which wrongfully reassure patients—and worst of all, produces many false positive results, which can cause terrible and damaging stress in otherwise healthy people. It is also expensive. All in all, if we look beyond the rationalizations, we might conclude that annual screening is a colossal waste of time, money and energy. In fact it is difficult to understand how as a society we could have persuaded ourselves that we could prevent cancer by using X-rays, which are known to be carcinogenic.

PAP SMEARS

Pap smears have become an integral part of our medical culture, and few people would question the diagnostic boon of the smear in picking up cervical cancer in its early stages. Yet in spite of widespread acceptance of the procedure, some disturbing questions remain.

The rationale for Pap smears is that there is likely progression of cervical changes which lead to invasive cancer; from normal cells, to atypical cells, to carcinoma-in-situ, to invasive cancer. With this assumption, the argument goes that intervention at an early stage in the proceedings will halt progression of the disease. However, the assumption itself is known to be incorrect, since nine out of ten abnormal Pap smears revert to normal spontaneously, but that has not stopped the widespread implementation of screening programs without any prior trials to demonstrate their efficacy.

A review of the Bristol Pap screening program, which started in 1966, concluded that screening may do more harm than good. Despite good organisation and a high population participation, the effect of screening on death rates was too small to detect. In the last five-year study period, in which approximately 200,000 women were screened, over 15,000 were told there was something abnormal on the smear, and some 6,000 were referred for colposcopy, in order to prevent a malignancy which would only occur in a handful of women. In other words, thousands of women were put through the agony of false positive test results, many with follow-up surgical intervention, for a disease they were never going to get anyway; and meanwhile the false negative rate was significant enough that those destined to get cancer seemed to get it anyway, somehow slipping through the screening process along the way. Even more sinister was the alarming increase in false positive calls, by staff who lived in fear of being held legally liable for false negative smears. The authors concluded that much of their efforts in the screening program was devoted to limiting the harm done to healthy women, and to protecting their staff from litigation.[4]

Clearly, it is dangerous to assume that Pap smear screening has no down-side when it may lead to unnecessary or ineffectual surgical intervention, post-surgical bleeding, difficulties with future pregnancies, difficulties with obtaining life insurance, and lasting worries about cancer.

Pap smears don't even appear to be effective in preventing mortality from cervical cancer. In many countries, the mortality has increased despite an intensive screening program; and in North America, where the mortality from cervical cancer may be declining, the decline started before the screening programs were put in place. Thus screening programs are probably redundant, but they are certainly not cheap. The cost of an office visit to have the test performed is about $25 and the cost of interpreting that test is about $11. It has been estimated that 40,000 smears and 200 excisional biopsies must be done, at a cost of at least a million dollars, for every life presumed to have been saved.

Meanwhile the periodic Pap ritual continues with many women having needless intervention based on the unquestioned assumption that "getting rid of it for once gets rid of it for good." However, such treatment may not in fact get rid of anything for good. Little thought is given to the possibility that if a pathological process is going on in the body, surgical ablation may well drive that process deeper.

In an extensive review of screening programs, *Canadian Family Physician* recommended continued screening, not because it did any good, but because its practice was so widespread that it would be difficult to admit it was useless. The Bristol study concurred, adding that it was essential for society never to introduce widespread unevaluated screening programs again.[5]

FETAL MONITORING

It has become standard practice in many maternity wards to use modern technology to monitor the progress of labour. Whereas in earlier days, the attending nurse would listen to the baby's heart rate every few minutes during the first and second stages of labour, today many obstetricians, family doctors and midwives use continuous electronic monitoring instead. Continuous monitoring is assumed to be superior to intermittent auscultation, and few physicians would disregard such a technological advance—especially under the very real threat of litigation following a birth with a poor outcome. Though several studies have shown that continuous fetal monitoring provides no advantage over traditional techniques even in high-risk pregnancies, the common assumption is that even if it does no good, at least it does no harm. Other studies, however, have indeed shown a related harm: low-risk pregnancies continuously monitored are more likely to end in Caesarean sections.

Some years ago *the Lancet* published an article reviewing eight studies on fetal monitoring, none of which showed any benefit from the procedure even in high risk pregnancies, but the article refused to condemn its use; and in spite of such evidence, it took almost ten more years before the Society of Obstetricians seriously considered changing its guidelines to reflect the study outcomes. Even so, to this day physicians and hospitals remain reluctant to switch off the monitors, citing expense, or a lack of experienced nursing staff as a reason to continue the practice. Scientific evidence it would seem, is not enough to over-ride the fear of malpractice suits.[6]

There is no doubt, however, that continuous fetal monitoring leads to trigger-happy obstetricians. There is a palpable tension in the air when the monitor is on, and everybody's eyes go to the machine when there is any indication that the baby's heart-rate has fallen, diverting attention from the mother at just the moment she needs it most. At the same time, the Caesarian section rate has topped 25% in many North American hospitals—a scandalously high intervention rate in a perfectly natural process. There can be little doubt that fetal monitoring is making a contribution to this state of affairs.

Once again, we see a technique designed as preventative producing an unfortunate side-effect. Physicians monitor because they are under enormous pressure to deliver a perfect baby and are afraid of being sued if they don't. Consequently, if there is the slightest indication that the baby is in any kind of distress, they opt for a Caesarean section rather than wait the situation out. When the section produces a normal baby, everyone congratulates one another for making a good decision, yet studies suggest that these babies were never in distress, and the section had been precipitated by doctors and patients becoming overly anxious.

HORMONE REPLACEMENT THERAPY (HRT)

It has become standard practice to recommend HRT for post-menopausal women to prevent the ravages of osteoporosis, and heart disease, regardless of whether as an individual they are at risk. Epidemiological studies suggest that prior to menopause, women seem to be protected from heart disease in a way that men are not; similarly, bone loss in women predisposed to it seems to accelerate after menopause. Studies have suggested that the use of HRT after menopause will reduce heart disease and fracture rates by as much as 50%.[7] On the face of it, then, it would seem prudent to prescribe HRT to everyone, as a preventative measure.

Closer examination of these studies however suggests that such conclusions may be premature, and the blanket prescription of HRT short-sighted. To begin with, most of the studies which suggested a reduction in heart disease were done with oestrogen alone (without the addition of progesterone), —a regimen which has been all but abandoned because of an unfortunate increased risk of endometrial cancer. The currently recommended regimens, which propose a combination of oestrogen and progesterone, have not actually been fully tested, and while they appear to alleviate the risk of endometrial cancer, there is a parallel concern that they may increase the incidence of breast cancer. Consequently, the use of HRT may be jumping from the frying pan into the fire.[8]

As for osteoporosis, physicians know it is best prevented by a good diet, daily exercise and not smoking. In other words, to use HRT to prevent what can be prevented by a woman's respect for and nurturance of her own body is not only missing the point, but is also exposing women to unnecessary risks.

Since most fractures from osteoporosis occur after age seventy-five, prevention requires that women use HRT over a long period of time—precisely the situation which produces maximum risk of breast or endometrial cancer. Furthermore, while women may use HRT enthusiastically for a year or two around their menopause to reduce troublesome symptoms, they will often stop using it afterwards, dissipating the preventative edge they may have gained against the loss of bone. Perhaps worst of all, to suggest that the medical establishment ought to prescribe and monitor older women's daily and risky hormonal supplementation over decades in the absence of symptoms smacks of a paternalism incompatible with an individual's experience of true health and healing.

Stated simply, the problem with HRT is this: *to reduce the risk of osteoporosis and heart disease, women should use HRT for as long as possible, while to reduce the risk of cancer, they should use it for as short a time as possible.* Thus, in spite of mountains of research, the physical evidence leaves women and physicians in a quandary, with no easy answer, unless they go beyond the strictly physical arguments to a deeper level, where they may find a more convincing argument against the use of HRT.

Most women's reproductive systems can be seen to go through three or four phases: pre-menarche/non-fertile, ovulating/fertile, menopausal, and post-menopausal/non-fertile. To artificially maintain women's bodies in an ovulating/fertile (pre-menopausal) state with HRT is to effectively prevent them from moving into the next stage of their lives: a stage that may constitute up to half of a woman's total lifespan, artificially trapping her body in the particular hormonal cycle relevant to fertility. We might question whether this kind of "entrapment" of women's bodies under the guise of a cure-all for the "hysteria" of menopause may be more a male need than a female one. For women who want to face the challenge of transformation and to explore themselves in a new stage of their lives, HRT may be a major stumbling block.

PROSTATE CANCER

It is currently recommended that after the age of forty men should undergo a digital rectal examination as part of their annual physical examination, the purpose being to detect prostate cancer, early enlargement of the prostate, ano-rectal cancer, or other ano-rectal problems. The hope seems to be that if prostate cancer could only be detected early enough, there would be a better chance of a cure. Recently a blood test called the "prostate specific antigen test," or PSA, has become popular as an adjunct to the digital rectal exam to pick up early prostatic carcinoma. Indeed, so popular has the test become that scarcely a day goes by in a doctor's office without someone requesting it, "just to be on the safe side." This concern is fuelled by statistics which show that prostate cancer is on the rise, that it is now the third leading cause of cancer death, behind colon and lung cancer and that only ten to twenty percent of prostate cancers are discovered early enough to be arrested. Indeed, so common is prostate cancer that it is probably present in half the population of men over eighty, though it may not cause them any trouble. Most of these elderly men will die of other causes, mercifully oblivious to the fact that they technically have a "prostate cancer".

It is not surprising that something so common if looked for will often be found; however, there is much debate as to whether diagnosing the disease has any real value. In fact, not only is there no good evidence that screening decreases mortality, but there is plenty that it *creates more medical problems*, related to both psychological stress and the surgical intervention which follows early detection. Patients can expect referral to a urologist, repeat rectal exam and PSA testing, trans-rectal ultrasound studies, followed by multiple needle biopsies, cystoscopy and X-rays. If a cancer is found they can expect radical surgery, radiotherapy, and possibly chemotherapy, with all the associated complications: pain, anastomotic leakage, incontinence, impotence, —all in spite of the fact that there is no change in overall mortality for those undergoing these procedures.

Several current reviews of screening methods have concluded that, given the lack of demonstrable benefit from screening and the significant associated morbidity, it is really unethical to screen for prostate cancer at all—with the digital test, the PSA, or anything else—unless the patient makes an informed decision, and accepts responsibility for the consequences. And that conclusion does not even take into consideration the enormous financial cost to society of the procedures, which is considerable.[9, 10, 11]

If patients were properly informed, it is hard to imagine them ever giving consent to a prostate examination. Unfortunately, the interpretation of various studies on the subject is so complex that virtually no one, physicians included, are sufficiently informed to leave the prostate well enough alone.

PREVENTION AND HOLISM

It is our contention that screening does not work because it is too narrowly focused and based on linear cause-and-effect thinking. That kind of thinking asks us to select only one or two end-points against which to measure the effectiveness of any given program. In this way, we justify accepting reduced cardio-vascular mortality for example, while ignoring the fact that overall mortality remains the same, or is even increased. The overall picture seems just too complicated, or irrelevant, and is therefore not studied. In fact, it isn't that complicated at all but quite straightforward and completely integrated, if seen holistically.

Linear thinking prevents us from accepting the results of even objective scientific studies at face-value—we feel that screening *must* have an effect, even when studies show none. On the other hand, holistic thinking, which considers disease an essential part of the healing response, would tell us quite the opposite: that prevention is at best useless and at worst likely to create more problems than it solves. In other words, *there probably isn't any beneficial effect from screening, even when it appears that there is.*

THE SIDE-EFFECTS OF SCREENING

The paradox of screening is that it appears to work but in fact does not, frequently leading to side-effects which may ultimately negate its benefits. If we look at these side-effects, we find that they fall into two groups, objective and subjective. It should come as no surprise by now that the objective side-effects are well recognized and justified, while the subjective consequences are hidden and denied.

OBJECTIVE SIDE-EFFECTS

Objective side-effects are simply the physical result of invasive intervention. Mammograms, for example, use X-rays which are known to be cancer-causing. The effect may be minute, but it is still there. Drug therapy, too, always produces side-effects, both short-term and long-term. For example, antibiotics upset the intestines, affect digestion and may lead to immune-system compromise. Those kinds of side-effects are both known and considered. They are seen to be bothersome, but acceptable.

SUBJECTIVE SIDE-EFFECTS

Subjective side-effects are emotional effects. Many patients are not particularly concerned about serious illness until the doctor mentions screening. Screening causes anxiety, as patients are naturally concerned that they might have a disease. Given that most of the diseases we screen for are the final manifestations of chronic anxiety, the fact that doctors knowingly *create* anxiety in their patients is one of the great ironies—not to say injustices—of our current medical system.

Obviously, then, any intervention which increases anxiety is working at cross-purposes—a fact almost never acknowledged by screening enthusiasts, as they are usually looking at disease from an entirely physical standpoint. That the psychological factors in the disease process, while well documented in many reputable studies, are not usually considered is actually not surprising. Those factors argue against prevailing prevention strategies, and to consider them would destroy the validity of all screening recommendations. For physicians and scientists who have given their lives to the objective ideal, to include the subjective nature of disease would entail a radical perceptual shift amounting to no less than a transformation.

PREVENTION AND PHILOSOPHY

A complete program of prevention must take both subjective and objective factors into consideration. Only then can we be sure that there are no hidden side-effects we have not considered. Before we can do this, however, we have to enlarge our understanding of illness to include the person who is ill. This idea is embedded in the traditional medicines of India and China. It also exists in our own Western tradition. Sir William Osler located the concept at the very heart of conventional medicine when he said, "The question is not what disease has the patient, but what patient has the disease."

So it's not that we haven't known all this before, it's just that we've lost many such central perceptions in our quest to sanctify objectivity. Osler's remark records his belief that individuals' personalities, lifestyles, diets, environment, work habits and beliefs all count in the diagnosis and treatment of their illnesses. He seems to have considered these factors more significant in the long run than whatever specific disease a patient was suffering from. Current preventative screening strategies are directed at the disease in question as though it existed in isolation, rather than at the person who may have the disease.

In fact, disease is not an "it." It is not a thing separate from other things. It does not exist by itself, but only in the context of the individual who has it. Disease is an expression of the state of an individual who has various symptoms. The separation of disease and patient exists in our imagination only, but is so embedded there that we operate as if this fantasy were a fact, and design our prevention and treatment programs around the idea of disease as independent entity. How can prevention strategies designed around such an erroneous assumption be expected to work? A program which emphasized people rather than disease would have to be structured very differently; and it is immediately obvious that screening programs that would take subjective factors into account would be far too complicated to be practicable.

PREVENTION AND TRANSFORMATION

The holistic perspective considers that anyone who is ill has a personality that has predisposed that individual to that illness. A "type-A" executive who smokes, works too hard, and never relaxes is prone to cardio-vascular disease. Prevention for that kind of person means more than just quitting smoking. Smoking is just another expression of his personality—as is any illness he might "attract." In fact, smoking, considered in isolation, might make him less anxious, and therefore less prone to illness. And even if he quits, the specific illness he might get will be different, but chances are he will still get ill.

Piecemeal prevention simply moves illness from place to place in the body, as studies often demonstrate. They note that overall mortality rates remain mysteriously unchanged without comprehending that their candidates, "saved" from one illness, simply died within the same period of another.

The inescapable inference of holistic thinking is that true prevention and healing are one and the same thing, and that real prevention must therefore involve healing of the total gestalt of the patient—mind, body, spirit and environment. An *effective* prevention program will therefore require the individual to embark on a transformational journey. In practice, however, the changes required are so great and so difficult that it often takes a serious illness to motivate us—at which point, if left alone, the imbalances we harbour reach a critical point, and transformative change occurs quite spontaneously, with the result that a more healthy person emerges.

Systems theory might predict such a process: when a system reaches a certain level of complexity and tension, it spontaneously changes to a higher level of organization. In other words, transformation is a normal, healthy and spontaneous process which occurs quite naturally throughout our universe when events are left to themselves. Any attempt to interfere with the process not only delays the change, but means that the change will be more violent when it occurs. From that perspective, all medical treatments based on maintaining our present gestalt are illness-producing, including all linear treatment and screening programs—and, paradoxically, illnesses which induce transformational change are health-giving.

THE PARADOX OF PREVENTION

Here we are up against a paradox again. It seems that the only way to have an effective prevention program is to allow people to get ill, and then resist the temptation to intervene, while we wait for the transformational journey to begin. Patients must get sick enough to want to change, but not sick enough to die.

Because of our cultural mind-set, well-meaning educational programs aimed at people who are not yet ill do not work very well. Nobody listens to advice unless they absolutely have to. We could stop spending millions on an outmoded health-care system which is bankrupting the nation, and start a collective transformational journey if we realized that. We could take information only to the places where it has a chance of being heard—to the young, and the chronically ill, to those individuals who have little investment in the status quo, and are willing to consider the prospect of change.

1. Psaty, B.M. et al. "The risk of Myocardial Infarction associated with Antihypertensive Drug Therapies"; *Journal of the American Medical Association*, August 23/30, 1995; 274:620-5.
   Buring, J.E. et al. "Calcium Channel Blockers and Myocardial Infarcation: a hypothesis formulated but not yet tested"; *Journal of the American Medical Association*, August 23/30, 1995; 274:654-5.
2. Wright, Charles J. et al. "Screening Mammography and Public Health Policy: The need for perspective"; *Journal of the American Medical Association*, Vol. 36, July 1, 1995; 29-32.
3. Glasziou, Paul., et al. "Mammographic screening trials for women aged under 50"; *The Medical Journal of Australia*, Vol. 162, June 19, 1995; 625-29.
4. Raffle, A.E. et al., "Detection rates for abnormal Cervical Smears: What are we screening for"; *the Lancet*; Vol. 345, June 10 1995, 1469-1473.
5. Satenstein, G. et al. "Consensus Statement from the Front Line"; *Canadian Family Physician*, Vol 37; October 1991; 2103-2115.
6. "Fetal Surveillance guidelines slammed" *Canadian Family Practice*, October 9 1995.
7. Canadian Menopause Consensus Conference; *Journal of the Society of Obstetricians and Gynecologists of Canada*; Vol 16, No. 5, May, 1994.
8. Colditz, G.A. "The use of Estrogens and Progestins and the risk of Breast Cancer in Post-Menopaulsal women". *The New England Journal of Medicine*, Vol. 332, No. 24, June 15, 1995; 1589-1593.
   Collins, J.A. "Hormone Replacement Therapy and Breast Cancer: What is Happening". *Journal of the Society of Obstetricians and Gynecologists of Canada*, Vol. 17, No. 9, September 1995; 837-849.
9. Marshall, Kenneth G. "Screening for Prostate Cancer"; *Canadian Family Physician*, Vol 39, November 1993; 2385-2390.
10. Cantor, Scott B., et al. "Prostate Cancer Screening: A Decision Analysis", *The Journal of Family Practice*, Vol. 41, No. 1 July 1995.
11. Budenholzer, Brian R. "Prostate Specific Antigen testing to screen for Prostate Cancer"; *The Journal of Family Practice*, Vol. 41, No. 3, September 1995; 270-78.

Chapter Sixteen

STRESS AND ILLNESS

Anxiety is good; an illness is better; a breakdown is best

*T*hrough understanding the relationship between accumulated inner stress and the development of disease, we can finally move beyond the present medical paradigm into the new age. When the connection between mind, body and spirit is fully established in our understanding, disease is no longer seen as a meaningless event. Should we wish to ignore the import of this connection individually, our present cultural imbalance is leading us inexorably toward its own transformation. The pressure building in our collective consciousness manifests itself daily in us as individuals as anxiety, stress and ultimately as disease. Two apparently quite different case histories will help us to illustrate the mind-body continuum and the connection between mental stress to physical illness.

JOAN

Joan was a thirty-six-year-old client with severe chronic back pain stemming from a trivial accident which occurred when she was eighteen. At the time, she had improved with the usual conservative treatments, but had had recurrent episodes of increasingly severe pain over the next twelve years. At the age of twenty-nine she was admitted to hospital for five weeks in such severe pain that she had to rest completely to get any relief. When she subsequently continued to have pain at home, she was diagnosed as having degenerative disc disease.

After some consideration of her options, Joan decided to take her doctor's advice and have surgery on two discs in her lower back. She was only thirty-one at the time.

Following the operation she felt relatively well until a minor injury, at age thirty-three, brought back all her pain. A this point, she was diagnosed as having arachnoiditis—an inflammatory condition affecting the nerve roots for which surgery is not effective—and was told that nothing further could be done. She began to take pain-killers in increasing quantities, and rapidly became addicted.

Slowly, the body-mind breakdown manifested itself in other ways, among them chronic fatigue and multiple food allergies. Predictably, she adopted a severely restricted diet, and spent a good portion of the day immobilized by her pain. By the time she came to see us she was in a wheelchair, her only other option being an operation to sever the sensory nerves in her spinal cord. Fortunately, some part of her knew that she should try something else and she decided to explore some alternatives before committing herself to such drastic surgery.

RICHARD

Richard was a hard driving forty-four-year-old chartered accountant, who considered himself in perfect health until he got an attack of 'flu while on vacation in Mexico at the age of thirty-nine. He never really bounced back from the illness as he was accustomed to do, and found himself feeling increasingly tired at work. He had difficulty waking up in the morning and getting out of bed.

As Richard was self-employed and felt that taking time off work was not feasible, he took to drinking coffee with sugar all day long to pep himself up, and a drink or two in the evening to help him get to sleep. At this point, he was diagnosed as having hypoglycaemia, and was advised to cut down on his intake of stimulants and sugar. He cut out his coffee and alcohol, reduced his intake of refined sugar, and for a few months he felt much better.

However, he soon began to develop allergies to other foods, responding with dizzy spells, nausea, and diarrhea. Eliminating these foods from his diet, however, made him feel even more tired. His doctor felt he might have "the Yeast Syndrome," and treated him with Nystatin, and dietary alterations. Again, he improved for a while, but when he stopped taking Nystatin his fatigue and allergies returned.

At this point, Richard got fed up. He gave up on doctors and began to take sleeping pills and tranquilizers to cope with his anxiety and insomnia. Again he felt better for a while. But soon his symptoms returned. In desperation, he gave the medical establishment another chance, and was diagnosed with Epstein-Barr virus disease.

At first he felt quite relieved at finding out what his problem really was, but at the same time found himself angry that the "real" diagnosis had been missed for so long. He joined an Epstein-Barr support group, where he met many other people with the same problem. After the first flush of relief at being surrounded by others who shared and understood his experience, he gradually realized that even with the support group, there was no solution in sight. One year later, his fatigue was no better and he was using increasing quantities of tranquilizers, both to help him to sleep and to manage his panic attacks. Finally, he was unable to work and came to our clinic.

THE PROBLEM OF ANXIETY

At first glance, the problems of these two individuals appear quite different. One situation involves an accident resulting in surgery and chronic pain. The other appears to be a viral infection. Yet these two patients have comparable histories when viewed from an energetic standpoint. Let's digress a little, take a look at anxiety from a cultural perspective, develop a working model, and then return to these particular cases to see what we can make of them.

One of the common experiences of our modern society is the chronic subliminal discomfort we all recognize as anxiety. It is such a familiar feeling to all of us that we tend to ignore it, deny it, and generally try not to think about it too much, for fear that focusing on it might make it worse.

The coupling of its general unpleasantness and its constant presence in the background of our experience has resulted in an anxiety-phobic culture. Yet, paradoxically, instead of doing something about it, we seem to gear our lifestyle to producing it in increasing quantities. In fact, the very fabric of our materialistic, industrial culture depends on *increasing* stress. Advertising surrounds us every day, in every conceivable place—on TV, in the newspapers, by the sides of our highways, on buses, t-shirts, in the supermarket aisles, and in elevators. There is nowhere we can go to get away from the constant pressure to consume, yet we are so accustomed to that we seems to think nothing of it.

Advertising generates anxiety in the consumer precisely in order to suggest that consumption will relieve it. There is no great secret about this strategy. The received wisdom is that in order to sell something, advertising must first demonstrate our need for it. Pharmaceutical companies have long capitalized on this market-creation technique to peddle their wares to the unwary, and it is interesting to note that some of the best money-makers in the business are the anxiolytics themselves. These drugs help curb the feelings of anxiety which are in part generated by pharmaceutical advertising. The problem and the solution are not so very different. Uncontrolled consumption is characteristic of a society in which everyone must go into debt in order to make a living. Indeed, society actively encourages us all to incur some debt in order to get a start in the world. University loans, borrowing to start a business, or having a mortgage on a house introduce us to life with a debt-load. In fact, debt is so ingrained in our culture that even our governments seem unable to do business without it. And all the while our collective anxiety keeps building.

The sad irony of it all is that we usually go into debt in order to buy long-term security, precisely to try to relieve that inner anxiety. We think that we will feel better if we have that reliable new car, or comfortable new house. Or we persuade ourselves that by investing wisely in our future we can purchase tomorrow's security. However we rationalize the compulsion, the fact is that the debt which we acquire through consumption may become one of the major problems which fuel our chronic inner tension. We find ourselves in a vicious cycle in which anxiety produces a desire to consume, which leads to acquiring debt, which leads to more anxiety—a pattern that can be traced in many other major causes of anxiety in our society, whatever their focus. The vicious cycle can be simply illustrated thus:

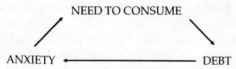

NEED TO CONSUME

ANXIETY ◄─────────────── DEBT

If we accept for a moment that anxiety is endemic, we see how the collective distortion manifests itself in the individual as disease and unease, or *dis*ease. By looking at the way the body reacts under the pressure of anxiety, we can see some very interesting parallels directly linking debt to tension. We know that the body under stress tightens up, and that the tightening results in the feeling of being anxious. We also know that the process is largely unconscious and goes on unnoticed. Most people will experience some tightening in their neck, back, or stomach when under stress, but few are aware of the hidden pressures which are generating their unease. The exact form of the tightening varies from person to person, and leads to a huge variety of stress-related symptoms, so that it takes a person with some insight to see beyond the superficial symptoms to the root cultural imbalance. Energy is required to maintain muscular tension, so with a little imagination we can look on tension patterns as a form of energy "debt" which strongly corresponds to monetary debt. In the case of acute stress such as a sports event or a public speaking engagement, the stress may be dealt with satisfactorily by the activity at hand, and the energy debt paid off. The body relaxes and tension patterns resolve—as though we'd paid off our credit card so that the balance was at zero.

Paying our accumulated "bills" relieves all manner of chronic tension and leaves us with much more freedom to manoeuvre, whereas unpaid energy debts require a continuous expenditure of energy to "service" them. Chronic anxiety or tension require us to throw good physical energy after bad. Furthermore, as we go through life absorbing more and more unresolved stress, our tension patterns accumulate it correspondingly. Initially, the energy we pay as interest on our stress is only a fraction of our total energy resources. If we are young and healthy, we can manage the debt easily. Because we have ample energy to spare, we don't necessarily even notice the gradual erosion of our energy capital. During the early stages of energy-debt behaviour, we are in a situation analogous to having a credit card with no upper limit, and an overspending habit which represents only a manageable portion of our income. We are fooled into thinking that we can go on forever, and so carry on expending energy rather unconsciously, not really looking too hard at the debt that is slowly piling up.

There is little doubt that most chronic tension patterns are unconsciously acquired in this manner, with little thought and even less conscious concern that we might be setting ourselves up for illness. Over time, however, we may find that our debt has built up to the point that we can make payments only on the interest and not on the capital; and finally we may barely be able to afford payments on the interest.

This losing battle is acted out in much the same way in the body. When we pay our energy debts promptly, our bodies remain in a precarious balance. Life carries on, but we may realize on some level that we are skating very close to the edge. It is a perilous existence with which many of us are very familiar. The ice underneath us threatens to crack at any moment, and when it does disease occurs. Just as there is a threshold above which interest payments become crippling, so there is a threshold for chronic tension above which symptoms of a disease process begin to surface. We are then at a point of no return, a point at which coping breaks down and the situation which generated the debt in the first place must be corrected.

Unfortunately, when disease or pain appears, the problem of energy debt becomes further compounded—our habitual tension itself is an extra stressor adding to anxiety and reducing the possibility of finding a simple solution.

THE STRESS-ILLNESS RELATIONSHIP

The development of chronic tension, or energy-debt, leading to illness conceptualized above indicates that disease does not just suddenly strike for no reason at all, but rather is the result of a long-accumulated, unresolved stress (*Figs. 1, 2, 3 & 4*).

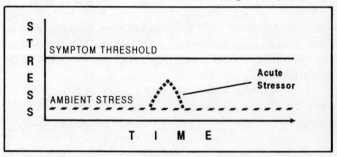

Fig.1—Stress and disease. Situation of low ambient stress.

In Figure 1, the model shows an individual with a low ambient stress level. Acute stressors come and go but do not trigger a symptom. Acute stressors can be anything that the body views as a problem—certain foods, alcohol, cigarettes, or marital tiffs. When we keep ourselves in this low ambient stress state, our lives are largely free of disease. We have adequate energy to go about our daily business and have little concern about developing any inter-current illness which may be going around.

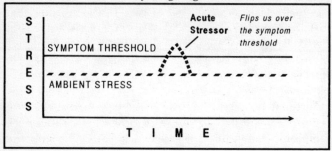

Fig. 2 — Stress and disease. Situation of high ambient stress

Figure 2 shows a life of high ambient stress. We feel OK most of the time, but will get sick when an acute stressor temporarily flips us above the symptom threshold. Someone who experiences a migraine after drinking red wine would likely be in this category. One regularly occurring acute stressor for women is the monthly period. From the model it is easy to see why some women are susceptible to pre-menstrual syndrome (PMS) or dysmenorrhoea during that time of extra stress. It is rather tragic that society does not acknowledge these conditions as precipitated as much by ambient stress as by hormones.

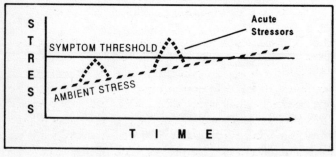

Fig. 3—Stress and disease. Situation of accumulating stress

In Figure 3, chronic stress has slowly built up, as it probably has done in most of us. Not only will an acute stress now eventually take us above the disease threshold, but even sustained ambient stress will take us on a crash course with illness. Because we are largely unaware of the process, we are taken by surprise and bewail our misfortune when we become ill. Illness has no meaning for us because we are not aware of our personal responsibility in the matter.

Fortunately, there is usually a significant period of time prior to a major breakdown during which we experience symptoms from acute stressors which would normally not bother us. If we take note of the various clues which indicate that our ambient stress is reaching a dangerous level, we can take steps to avoid misfortune before an overt pathological process develops.

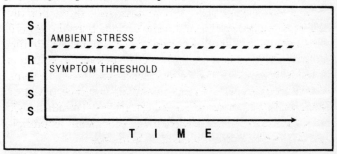

Fig. 4—Stress and disease. Situation of pathological stress.

In Figure 4, the chronic stress level is very near or even above the disease threshold. In this situation, we may well be ill all the time. Unfortunately, such chronic illness is becoming all too common in modern society because so few recognize the significance of this state of constant stress. When illness develops in this way it is always chronic in nature, and it may take almost any conceivable form, but its common feature is its complete resistance to any form of conventional therapy. In fact, if an illness does not respond to conventional treatment, then stress is very likely to blame. Further, given that the illness is ultimately a result of overload, and given that medical intervention is often very stressful, conventional therapy can make the problem worse. Reversing this scenario indicates that we will be more successful if we tap directly into our own resources and connect ourselves to the strength that is within us.

INVERSE RELATIONSHIP OF STRESS AND ENERGY

It is reasonable to assume that many people in our society have unacceptably high ambient stress. These people are therefore functioning close to the disease threshold all the time. When they eventually flip over the threshold, we can predict the kind of illnesses they will get.

It's not difficult to see that chronic stress and energy must be inversely related. When the body is severely stressed, the resulting chronic tension uses up all the available energy, and the body's total energy decreases accordingly. Finally, at the threshold for disease, all available body energy is totally exhausted.

Let's look now at some possibilities:

Food allergies appear. The digestive system requires energy to do its job. When there is little energy, the body cannot digest the food which it takes in. Clinical ecologists have postulated that allergies appear when the digestive system does not break down food completely and foreign proteins are absorbed unchanged into the body. Since the body is not meant to deal with foreign protein, it reacts as if the food were an allergen. If elimination diets are used at that point, the patient will in all likelihood become nutritionally deprived, making the problem of low energy worse.

Frequent infections. The immune-system requires energy if it is to function properly. When there is no energy, the body becomes open to infection from a variety of otherwise harmless agents (e.g. the common cold, Epstein-Barr virus and Candida). We could speculate that even AIDS may fit into this low-energy category.

Chronic fatigue. Exhaustion is the direct experience of a low energy state.

Poor mental functioning. The brain requires a high energy supply to function properly, hence low energy results in mental difficulties. One aspect of poor mental functioning is insomnia, which is a very common experience when we are highly stressed. When sleep is disturbed, this adds stress to the system, maintaining the imbalance. Without sufficient sleep, the energy deficit increases and cannot be spontaneously corrected.

THERAPEUTIC OPTIONS IN STRESS-INDUCED ILLNESS

We can see in the various diagrams that there are at least three possible ways of dealing with stress-induced illness. Two tactics involve controlling symptomatology, and a third deals with underlying tension patterns.

1/ *Treat each symptom as it arises.* Even though conventional medicine prides itself on thoroughness and a rigorous search for the root cause of an illness, emphasis is always placed on the search for a physical or biochemical cause. Since the root cause of illness is often at a deeper level than the physical (i.e. the root cause is mental or spiritual), the net result of this approach is symptom suppression. If this remark sounds extreme, consider the previously mentioned situation in which someone develops a migraine after drinking red wine. Conventional medicine holds that migraines result when certain vaso-active substances are released which cause arteries in the brain first to contract, then to expand. The release of the chemicals may be facilitated by a trigger substance such as red wine, cheese, or anything to which one may be sensitive, so that the entire process is explained biochemically. Stress factors are accorded some influence, but they are not seen as "causal." Given this mechanistic explanation, logic dictates that the appropriate treatment for migraine would be drugs which interfere with the mechanism. The result is that the headache is treated, but not the underlying stress, which is the deeper root cause. And the same reasoning applies in many other illnesses.

2/ *Avoid triggers*. Clinical ecology is a relatively new field of study which lies in the fringe area between conventional and alternative medicine. Using a variety of methods, practitioners seek to discover environmental sensitivities or allergies by observing the influence of a particular substance on the patient's electro-magnetic field. When a sensitivity is found, patients are advised to avoid that particular food or substance. While avoidance of such triggers makes good sense when there are only one or two particular food sensitivities, it makes less sense when there are multiple sensitivities, because avoidance of many kinds of foods simply leads to poor nutrition. Unfortunately, multiple sensitivities are becoming common as more and more people try to cope with high levels of ambient stress, and the nutritional deprivation which results from the clinical ecology approach simply makes the situation worse. Once again, such treatment is not reaching the root of the problem, but only dealing with physical manifestations or symptoms.

3/ *Pay attention to the unresolved tension patterns*. The new medicine looks beyond the physical expression of disease to its mental and spiritual roots. The treatment of physical symptoms is seen as only part of the greater picture which needs to be understood for true healing to occur. A holistic approach to a migraine syndrome might indeed advise the avoidance of trigger foods, for instance, while at the same time focusing on the deeper issues of stress and anxiety which are contributing to the overall situation. De-stressing techniques can reduce ambient stress to a level at which food sensitivities begin to disappear and headaches cease.

BREAKDOWN AND TRANSFORMATION

Anxiety and stress have been increasing so rapidly in our culture that it has now reached epidemic proportions. Many of us are living close to the disease-threshold all the time. Physicians estimate that up to ninety percent of the illnesses they see in an average day are rooted in chronic anxiety. And whether they realize it or not, the traditional approach of calming the anxiety with drugs does nothing but put off the day of reckoning. Also on the increase are people with chronic immune system dysfunction—reflected in such diverse conditions as multiple allergies, chronic infections, chronic fatigue, and possibly AIDS.

There is little doubt that our culture has reached a stage of high ambient stress. The body-mind of the cultural matrix has started to break down and the anxiety of many individuals within it only reflects a greater malaise. Breakdown is inevitable in a society living with a chronic energy debt. Many of us are getting sick in ways which defy rational therapy, leaving us little recourse but to explore our own mental and spiritual resources. In this way, a cultural transformation is subtly occurring. Illness has become the threshold of a new way of living—a way of living in greater awareness. And given that illness is almost inevitable, the most creative choice we have to make is to begin our own transformative journey.

It seems that the best type of breakdown to have, the most health-giving one in the long run, is that which might be called a break*through*—one which spares the physical body so that full recovery is possible. Mental breakdown is unfortunately associated with mental hospitals, social ostracism and lifelong illness and so strikes terror into many people. Much more common however is the so-called "nervous breakdown" in which chronic anxiety has reached a crisis point, and the person can no longer function. This sort of breakdown usually spares the body and can initiate the transformative journey from breakdown to breakthrough.

Breakdown to breakthrough characterizes both cases presented at the beginning of this chapter. For one reason or another both patients had exhausted their reserves of energy and were developing more and more symptoms, none of which seemed amenable to rational or conven-

tional solutions. Stress, anxiety and illness are so inti-
mately related that it is ultimately impossible to separate
them. If we are willing to learn the lessons inherent in the
experience of stress and anxiety we, like the Green
Knight, can speed our journey to our appointment with
destiny and reach a state of super-wellness. Through
transforming our fundamental outlook, the energy which
is locked up in chronic tension patterns can be released,
and healing can occur in all dimensions of our being.

Chapter Seventeen

ACCIDENTS AND METAPHYSICS

An accident is no accident

$\mathcal{A}$ccidents are a major source of chronic pain and illness and over the years we have seen literally hundreds of accident "victims" of one kind or another. One thing that has struck us as most odd is no one who has an accident ever feels that they had anything to do with it. Accidents just seem to happen to people—the "victim" feels totally innocent.

Is it possible that people who cause, say, automobile accidents rarely hurt themselves? Or do they hurt themselves but not come for treatment? We don't think so. Much more likely is that a group of people who are feeling particularly victimized by circumstance are manifesting some amount of denial. After all nobody *wants* an accident—or at least nobody *thinks* they want an accident. Certainly, an accident by definition isn't planned. They are unexpected, but may involve factors we don't care to admit to ourselves.

One of the ideas which seems to permeate "New Age" thinking is the notion that "we attract that which occurs to us." Nothing is more irritating to the average scientific mind than that particular "causal" explanation of events. It seems that the metaphysician wishes to ascribe causality where no causality can exist. What's more, the idea seems to lay the blame with us for the disagreeable events in our lives. It is bad enough to have an accident or to get ill. If we must also accept that we somehow attracted our mis-

185

fortunes, we have to add guilt to the burden of sickness and pain.

Laying blame is not the intent of such a belief. Instead, it suggests a restoration of the sense of personal power which an accident, if seen as a "victimizing" necessarily removes. This sense of personal responsibility, in the sense of power, not blame, is the fuel of the transformational journey. If we could step back and observe the high ambient stress we all carry, it would be easy to understand the reasoning behind the "attraction" principle of metaphysics.

At the disease or symptom threshold a breakdown of one sort or another is inevitable. The threshold is in essence an "event horizon," a point at which something is bound to happen. When there is high ambient stress, the mind becomes absorbed in all the problems which are assaulting it, so has little energy left to focus attention on the present moment. More and more of our attention is taken up in worrying about the various things which are going on in our lives, with the inevitable result that attention is diverted from immediate events. If attention to the present moment is reduced for whatever reason, then the probability of an accident must be increased.

Our society seems to have chosen to battle drinking and driving with an alarming single-mindedness, as though alcohol were the only thing which compromises our attention. We are all familiar with the statistics which link the consumption of alcohol to accidents, so it should not be difficult to appreciate the idea that the phenomenon is a direct result of reduced attention to the present moment. If alcohol-induced distraction affects a driver, we can see by extension how many other factors can and do contribute to compromised perception in just the car environment alone. Attention can be reduced by talking on a car phone, smoking, prescription or other drugs, preoccupation with stressful events, bee stings, kids in the back seat, or any similar distraction. When we are on the verge of burn-out, when we are at or near the symptom threshold, we are in a sense an "accident waiting to happen" or an "illness waiting to occur."

The essential point here is that while accidents are accidents, they cannot be fully explained without reference to the states of consciousness of the people involved. When an event occurs with more frequency than would be normally expected, it can certainly appear that an "attractive" force is at work, "making" the event take place. Whether there is actually any force, or only the appearance of one, is probably as much a matter of semantics as it is of fact.

For example, when dice are thrown repeatedly, the number seven comes up more often than any other number. One way of explaining why that happens is that there is a "force" which is making the dice come up with sevens. The explanation of "statistical probability" is, after all, simply teleological. Our observation of the *appearance* of a force gives us permission to describe the phenomenon that way: we can say that the dice "attract" the number seven because that's what they seem to do—that's what we see them do. To change the statistical probability that any particular number would come we could weight the dice slightly. By doing so, we could change the nature of the "force," and direct it to a number other than seven, creating a situation in which the nature of the dice themselves become a factor in the calculation of probabilities.

We assume that all dice are created equal, of course. Under normal circumstances we are no doubt correct. But if we tinker with the dice, we tinker with the probabilities. In the world of car accidents a similar interplay of factors is going on. Accidents are accidents, perhaps, but the increasing number of cars on the road naturally increases the frequency of accidents—the more cars, the more car accidents. People are driving the cars, and people unlike dice have individual "weights," or states of awareness, related to who they are and what is going on in their lives.

Insurance companies are well aware of individual differences as they try to assess relative risks for different groups of people. So far the best they have been able to do is to base risk on age and sex. However, so many people think risk groups are unfair that in some places another approach has been adopted: everyone is assumed to have the same risk until they actually have an accident, at which point they are deemed to be a higher risk—and many insurance companies refuse to back up a claim if the driver has increased the risk of an accident by drinking.

The concept of "risk groups" clearly supports the idea that different people have different states of consciousness, which may or may not predispose them to accidents. From that point of view, the idea that we "attract" accidents to us is no great mystery but merely an observation of the fact that under certain conditions, certain people will have more accidents. At this point whether we say that people are prone to accidents, or that accidents are prone to them seems academic.

The various factors which lead people to be "accident prone" can also be described as body-mind "stressors"—and these can be anything which demands our attention and energy. Present attention becomes compromised resulting in a decrease of "consciousness in the moment," which in turn results in the greater probability of an accident.

Accidents therefore are accidents, but they are also not accidents. They are expressions of the totality of our state of consciousness. In particular, they are expressions of the levels of ambient stress which we carry. What's more, accidents themselves add a further stressor to a system which is already highly stressed. It is a disturbing feature of accidents that many people involved in them are at or near the symptom threshold without knowing it at the time of their accident. Predictably, in these cases the additional stress of the accident may push such people permanently over the symptom threshold into the syndrome of chronic pain.

All this is not to say that accidents never occur to people with low levels of ambient stress. They do. These people, however, are much less likely to go on to develop chronic

David L

ls.

spa.

ennis courts,
our pools.
e from

k/april

nal fees.
isure on a
ldren will need to
ear old standalone
day pass

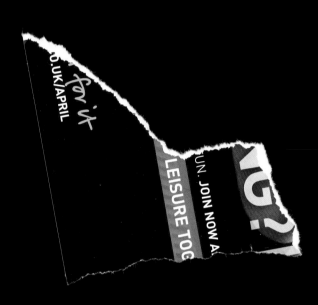

pain. They are the ones who get better in six to eight weeks and carry on with their lives. Others may be so disturbed—or served —by the same accident that they seem unable to recover at all.

SECONDARY GAIN

When we first started treating patients with chronic pain, we noticed that people tended to have accidents or get ill during the course of the program just at the moment they began to relax chronic tension patterns. Eventually, in fact, as the meaning of these incidents became clear to us, we would begin to question whether they were getting anything out of the treatment if neither occurred. On the surface, expecting accidents or illness to occur during therapy seems a very strange thing. But let's look further.

Accidents, as we have seen, are likely to occur when we are burned out. When we are burned out, what we need more than anything else is time to reassess our situation and look for creative solutions. That and rest. Given that most of us would think it unacceptable to walk away, even briefly, from our problems, however onerous; then, an accident—and often *only* an accident, or serious illness— can possibly provide the "legitimate" breathing space we need. Indeed, there is often *so* much to gain by having an accident or becoming ill, that some people get stuck at the accident stage and forget to look for a solution.

In our society, accident or illness provides both a reason for rest, and the financial security necessary to supply everyday needs and fulfil our responsibilities. Insurance covers our mortgage payments, and feeds our kids, while our illness or accident earns us the respect, sympathy, and help of family and supporters. This is the paradox of "secondary gain"—the enormous positive value of illness and accidents, which we have great difficulty admitting to ourselves, let alone anyone else, protecting ourselves from such guilty truths behind a cloak of denial so thick that only the brave dare to penetrate it.

The principle of "attraction" might in this instance be recast as "we get what we need"—we attract not only what we fear but what we need to attract. Not only are we an accident waiting to happen, when we live with high levels of stress, but a part of us actually *wants* the accident because of the secondary gains it offers. In this context, people who have an accident during a treatment program reveal that they still need the pain or incapacity which brought them into the program. They are approaching the point of transformation, the critical moment when they have to deal with the reason they are ill. The accident gives them another reason to avoid making the change.

Only when we can clearly acknowledge what the accident or illness is doing for us can we start to solve our problems directly. If, for example, an illness gets us more attention and recognition, then if we wish to heal we must learn to ask for the recognition directly, rather than indirectly through illness.

ACCIDENTS AND DENIAL

Perhaps the most difficult part of the healing process for accident victims is taking the monumental step required to lift this cloak of denial. When we ask patients with chronic pain to list their secondary gains they often look at us as though we were out of our minds. Yet without probing that question the healing process remains completely blocked. To admit to ourselves that we have attracted our misfortunes is to move to a new state of responsibility in which we acknowledge the strength we all possess to effect our own destiny.

The difficulty is, secondary gain is often obvious to everyone dealing with the chronically ill except the patients themselves. Talk to any group of insurance adjusters about chronic pain. You'll find they're convinced that most accident victims are deliberately malingering—and many physicians feel the same way. After a while, there is a noticeable tension in the air when these patients interact with professionals. Patients feel invalidated in what to them is a very real experience, and professionals feel totally frustrated dealing with people who are both hostile and seemingly malingering. As none of them may be fully aware of the dynamics of feeling and denial, such situations can remain subconscious and hidden.

The conflict which lies beneath the cloak of denial is taboo. But before we can heal ourselves we have to confront it and the denial which clothes it. Until the benefits of illness are recognized and alternate means of achieving them worked out, we will not be ready to heal. We have to fully recognize the paradoxical truth that accidents are not accidents, and that illnesses are present because we need them. It is just not possible to get better otherwise. To heal from within requires that we see illness as a choice, a way to solve the unsolvable, and with that understanding move on to a creative solution.

Chapter Eighteen

MEDICINE AND
THE POWER STRUGGLE

Knowledge is ignorance; not knowing is wisdom

$\mathcal{T}$he link between consciousness and disease has been recognized by many philosophers over the years. Why is it that society as a whole does not recognize it? Why is it that so many people are unable to take personal responsibility when they become ill? These are not easy questions to answer. For some reason, it seems that as a culture we have yet to grow up and embrace adult responsibilities. We seem stuck in the rebelliousness of youth, struggling against things instead of moving with them.

The work ethic, the struggle to achieve and get to the top are examples of this sort of adolescent behaviour—reflecting an image of life as a constant power struggle. But buying in to a life of power struggles is not the only way to live. Such struggles are simply a stage in our development, prior to transformation, during which denial has the upper hand.

In Chapter 14, we discussed the existence of the barrier against the new medicine, and showed how breakthrough could be facilitated by the use of breathing techniques. We also talked earlier about the process of shifting perspectives and likened it to turning over a dollar bill. In this chapter, we want to focus a little more closely on the nature of the power struggle itself, in order to shed more light on the great difficulties which the confrontation produces both in our individual and collective experience. The struggle has been alluded to by many authorities using many different metaphors, and applied to many areas of human experience. Here we want to use mythology to show how the concept can be applied specifically to illness and healing.

THE CALIPH AND THE MENDICANT

One day, when the caliph was in his court receiving petitioners, a mendicant came in and offered him an apple. The caliph graciously accepted the gift as was his wont, but noted that his visitor said nothing by way of explanation. Without much more ado, then, he gave the apple to his treasurer and asked him to look after it. The royal chancellor, whose position gave him a keen awareness of the worth of things, tossed the mere fruit without ceremony into the storehouse with all the other royal offerings. The next day, however, the same strange visit was repeated; and thereafter every day for ten years. In time, the caliph got quite used to the daily visits of the silent mendicant who arrived in his court every day at the same hour, and gave the caliph his apple without petition, asking for nothing, saying nothing. The caliph, in his turn, passed the apple on to his treasurer who tossed them with increasing irritation into an unused area of the palace storeroom.

Strange things happen in a caliph's court, and one day a monkey happened to be in the room in which the caliph received his petitioners. The beggar arrived as usual for his daily visit, but just as the caliph was passing the apple to his treasurer, the monkey snatched it away and began to eat, causing a ripple of suppressed laughter to spread through the room. Suddenly however the amusement turned to amazement as a large jewel fell to the ground from the core of the fruit and lay at the monkey's feet, dazzling in the light.

The caliph was intrigued at this unexpected occurrence, and when he could get nothing out of the mendicant by way of explanation, asked his treasurer what happened to all the other apples. The treasurer explained that he had tossed them through a window into the back of the storehouse, and hurried off at the caliph's behest to have a look. A few minutes later the goggle-eyed and breathless man returned to describe the extraordinary hill of precious stones the ten-year-old mound of fruit had rotted into.

All of a sudden, the caliph was very eager to talk to his silent visitor, but during the commotion the strange little beggar had taken the opportunity to slip away. All was not lost, however. The next day at his usual hour, the old beggar appeared with another piece of fruit which he offered to his caliph.

He found the caliph eager for discussion. What was the meaning of all the jewels in the fruit? The old man must want something, surely. The beggar nodded gravely; yes, there was something he wanted; whereupon the caliph swore that if it were within his power to grant it, he would.

The mendicant then explained. Breaking his ten year silence, he said that needed the caliph to help him with the ritual he would be performing at midnight the following night on the execution hill above the city. The caliph had to be alone.

The next evening, following his instructions, the caliph dressed in simple clothes to disguise himself and climbed up the execution hill to meet the beggar. The old man was dressed in quite different garb, something akin to a priest's smock. He asked the caliph to cut down one of the many corpses which were hanging from the gallows and bring it across to a clearing where he had made a circle of stones.

Taken aback, but intent on honoring his pledge, the caliph nervously crossed the hill, cut down a corpse and, putting it over his shoulder, started to walk back to the circle. To his horror, the body he staggered to carry over the loose stones of the hillside began to address him. It said, "I am going to pose a riddle to you. If you know the answer and say something I will fly back to the gallows. If on the other hand you know the answer but say nothing your head will explode."

The caliph was by now so committed to the strange proceedings that he decided to take everything in his stride and instructed the spectre to carry on. He knew the answer the first riddle and had to speak; and, as promised, the corpse flew back to the gallows. Following his odd companion back to his execution site, the caliph once again cut down his corpse down and started walking across the hill, only to have it tell him another riddle to which he knew the answer.

This process continued most of the night until the caliph was totally frustrated and exhausted. He had promised the mendicant his help in the ritual, but in spite of all his efforts, he was unable to get his corpse over to the circle so that they could start. The beggar did not seem to be at all concerned, however, and was waiting quite patiently for the caliph to complete his task. After what seemed like an eternity, the spectre finally posed a riddle the caliph couldn't answer. Sighing with relief, he continued on his way across to the circle. But just as he approached the circle the spectre spoke again, warning him that the ritual to be performed was in fact his own execution and detailed the whole procedure. He told the caliph that the mendicant would ask him to do various acts of obsequiousness to his corpse, and finally to prostrate himself and kiss the ground. At that point the caliph's head would be chopped off.

The caliph completed his journey and placed the corpse in the centre of the circle as he was instructed. When he had done it, the mendicant began singing in a low voice and muttering strange things, all the while appearing perfectly composed and confident. Meanwhile, the caliph knelt before the corpse and witnessed the proceedings with a mixture of fear and exhilaration.

When the mendicant finished his ritual and asked the caliph to do a full obeisance to the corpse, the ruler knew it was time to act or die. Feigning ignorance, the wily ruler asked the mendicant to demonstrate exactly what he had to do so that he would not make a mistake. When the old beggar agreed and bent down to kiss the ground, the caliph seized the opportunity to turn the tables, and chopped off the beggar's head. The caliph returned to the palace a changed man.

The haunting story above beautifully illustrates the difficulties of the power struggle stage in our lives. So, before interpreting the story itself, let's take a moment to define this stage. In the journey we all must undertake toward healing, the stage of the power struggle is a stopping place, a point beyond which many people will not venture because to go beyond it means confronting our worst fears and submitting to the annihilation of a phase transition. In her book, *Couples Journey: Intimacy as a Path to Wholeness*, Susan Campbell describes the various stages through which a marriage relationship passes (*fig. 1*). First comes the romantic stage when the couple first meets and falls in love. At that point everything seems wonderful, magical. At this stage we role-play to please our partner, pretending to be someone we are not. We hope that by assuming this role we will be able to have the relationship we want.

Shortly, however, most relationships move to the stage of the power struggle. At this point we begin to realize that things are not exactly the way we thought they would be. We begin to think we may have made a big mistake. The very things that first attracted us to our partner now begin to rub us the wrong way, and we fight back with a variety of manipulative techniques learned in childhood in an attempt to alter their behaviour. They at the same moment of course are more than likely doing the same to us.

This struggle for control can turn a relationship into more of a war than a partnership, until every remark and gesture seems a tactical manoueuvre. Techniques of manipulation have no place in an adult relationship, and step by step, anger and resentment take the place of love. Paradoxically, however, the very disillusionment which makes our relationship seem a disaster, can also be a threshold, an opportunity. Disillusionment can in fact show us the way out of our power struggles. By literally "de-illusioning," us, it forces us to see life anew, to stand in the present moment, and to dispense with outmoded feelings and ideas, some of which may date far back into our childhood and are no longer appropriate. This new understanding can lead to a period of stability in our relationships in which we begin to work together. Co-creation, the final stage, occurs when we stop seeing our partner as separate from ourselves.

Life is about relationships, whether they are with different people, with a disease, or with ourselves. Ultimately, it is about a relationship between the self, or subject, and something or someone else, our object(s). Just as the physicists of earlier decades realized they could not describe the world/object as separate from the observer/subject, so too must we find the resolution of our relationships through discovering ourselves rather than trying to control.

Power struggles are an attempt to manipulate the objective world while ignoring our own subjectivity—a difficult, ultimately impossible task. Such opposition can only end when we are willing to dissolve the distinction between ourselves and the other. Several authors have described similar staging processes while discussing other kinds of relationships. In *On Death and Dying*, Elisabeth Kubler-Ross talks of our relationship with death, and points out various stages in the dying process; and Scott Peck in *The Road Less Travelled* describes four stages in the relationship with self on the spiritual journey. By listing these stages side by side we can begin to see the similarity between them all.

· CAMPBELL— marriage	· KUBLER-ROSS —death	· PECK—spiritual development
· Romance	· Denial	· Anarchy
· Power struggle	· Anger	· Fundamentalism
· Stability	· Bargaining	· Cynicism
· Commitment	· Despair	· ——
· Co-creation	· Acceptance	· Mysticism

Figure 1—Comparison of the various stages of relationship between the "self" and "other" by three different authors. Susan Campbell: marriage, Elisabeth Kubler-Ross: death, and Scott Peck: spirit.

Each author describes a stage of struggle which is resolved by disillusionment, by despair, or by surrender. The "bargaining" which Kubler-Ross describes is essentially no different from the struggle we engage in with our partners to make them change, and the fundamentalism of the spiritual seeker is in the same category. Fundamentalist thinking establishes its own moral rightness by making others wrong, and sees the solution to the world's problems in converting others to its particular path. When we try to impose our views on other people, we are engaging in a power struggle.

The stages which apply to a personal or spiritual relationship are exactly the same as the stages of our relationship with illness. We engage in the power struggle when we try to make our disease go away, or if we try to suppress it with drugs. Our unquestioned assumption that illness is something bad and should be removed is in fact a fundamentalist assumption that something is bad if we do not like it. The ensuing logic in both cases dictates a struggle designed to root out evil.

MYTHOLOGY AND THE POWER STRUGGLE

Let's take another look at our story to see how it describes the process of struggle, disillusionment and healing. As human beings we often appear to be comfortable—often, like the caliph, quintessentially so—on the surface, but there is always a mild irritant or nagging doubt in the mind that all is not right, that perhaps there is more to life than appearances suggest. The beggar's silent, enigmatic presence in the early scenes of our story might be seen as representative of such "background anxiety."

But just as the fruit is thrown into the treasury, the jewels within unnoticed, the meaning of the beggar's visits, like the meaning of our anxiety goes unexamined. For years and years the comfortable self ignores the beggar's silent proddings, and the conscious self sees no meaning in his gifts. Chance, like a monkey, comes along and produces a serious illness, and suddenly we see in the everyday gift of health we'd taken for granted a jewel of inestimable worth. And so we go after the physician and ask him the secret of his knowledge.

The caliph was so keen on finding the secret of the jewels, that he blindly submitted himself to the beggar's ritual without questioning the man's intent. Similarly, the patient wants the health promised by medicine and so follows the physician's instructions without question. The decision to surrender power to in order to receive the benefits of the physician's presumed knowledge sets the patient on a dangerous path of submission in the blind belief that the medical profession has all the answers.

The caliph chose to submit himself to the whims of the beggar, and found himself trying to carry out a task for which all his royal training and knowledge proved a hindrance—the very image of the power struggle we typically engage in to rid ourselves of illness. By following the beggar's instructions, the caliph found himself on execution hill carrying a corpse which spoke to him in riddles.

Illness likewise sits heavily on our backs like a corpse—
our own corpse: the very image of the death we fear.

Equally, every time we think we've answered its demands, proved ourselves equal to its riddles, and have
found a way to get better, our disease has a nasty habit of
returning, refractory to treatment, or turning up in another form. It is only when we run out of answers that the
real solution appears. Once the caliph passes the hurdle
of the riddles, he receives the most profound message of
all: if he carried on blindly in the ritual he would be killed.

The caliph's reaction to the beggar represents the fantasy we all have that someone or something is going to
come along and save us from our ills. We all hope for the
miracle cure, or magic bullet promised by scientific medicine. But by being quite literally forced to listen to the
body he is bearing through the night towards his own
death, the caliph finally understands, unmasks and
"beheads" his cherished self-delusions, freeing himself
from their bondage.

But he only does so when it comes to a question of kill
or be killed. When as patients we blindly follow professional advice, we are often told to go the hospital or clinic
where we are asked to participate in a series of tests and
treatments, the meaning of which is known only to the
physicians themselves. Thus begins the ritual of modern
medicine. Meanwhile, our bodies talk in riddles to us as
we struggle to do what the doctor has asked. Like the
caliph returning to the corpse, we keep repeating a futile
exercise, returning repeatedly to one physician or another, but never quite finding a solution. Nothing fundamental changes until we realize that there is no rational
answer to the problem which illness poses. With this realization comes huge relief, the sort of relief the caliph felt
as he finally succeeded in getting his body across the hill,
albeit that much closer to his death.

Paradoxically, if we despair and give up hope of cure,
suddenly the greater riddle is solved. At this moment,

the caliph's body unequivocally informs him that as he crosses the hill he is in fact going towards his own death. Immediately, he realizes that only he can save himself. That moment of self-realization is the moment of transformation, the beginning of the end of the power struggle, the point of *dis*-illusionment, and the point of entry into the phase transition. With disillusionment comes an incredible insight—the constant search for cause is part of the problem. Solution and cause are the same, and we realize that we must end our unquestioning dependence on the superficial remedies of traditional medicine if we truly want to heal.

When we realize that our delusions about the power of the medical system, with its promise of easy health, may be part of the problem of illness, we are willing to abandon those illusions and give ourselves over into our own care. After all, as in the story, we have to kill the beggar or die. Unfortunately, the power struggle is so compelling it is difficult to get beyond it. Our cultural consciousness is rooted in an adversarial system and our institutions are founded on it, so that we often live our whole lives immersed in a way of thinking which is ultimately destructive.

Not surprisingly, the impact of power struggles are everywhere in evidence around us. Not only is this kind of struggle involved in producing individual disease, but is destructive of the earth itself. Man's struggle against nature—ironically, the very definition of "civilization" through the ages—now threatens the survival of the planet. And, significantly, all our struggling to arrest our global ills has only led us deeper into trouble. In many ways, the solution has become the problem. The planet is in the same predicament as the individual who is facing chronic illness—there is no solution except to despair and to transform.

Chapter Nineteen

DARK NIGHT OF THE SOUL

Paradise found is paradise lost

*M*any times we have seen patients appear to heal, or undergo a major transformational experience, only to watch the euphoria wear off and see them crash into a depression far worse than anything they have known before. Often it seems that the greater the healing experience, the greater the crash. Just when everything seems heavenly, all hell breaks loose.

A sudden transformative experience is an awesome thing to witness. The shift in an individual's perception of the world is a truly momentous event. As witnesses to such an event, we can easily be misled into thinking that the transformation represents a complete healing. The drama of the change is so impressive that we can forget that shifts in perception can be slow as well as fast.

Transformation does not have to be a sudden event. It can take the form of subtle shifts over a period of time, and in fact when it does happen slowly, it is more likely to be stable. A simple analogy can be found in the shifting plates of the San Andreas fault line. A sudden large adjustment produces a more or less devastating earthquake. A lot of smaller shifts on the other hand can achieve the same release of pressure over time—without an accompanying cataclysm. This analogy is worth remembering when working with someone who is struggling with a healing process. Sudden revelations are miraculous to be sure, but they are not necessarily the only way to go.

THE TRANSFORMATIONAL CRISIS

Sometimes, in fact, it is best not to heal too fast, as the price of rapid success may be devastation. Paradoxically, the best results often occur when people do not seem to progress very quickly initially yet get enough to give them some direction for the future.

When transformation is sudden, the psyche may not be able to integrate the new information, and the conflict introduced may be unresolvable. The immediate presence of a new, contradictory apprehension of the world can result in profound psychological confusion which appears to destroy the gains which have been made. Clearly, we need to understand the process in order not to be stopped short. In its extreme form, transformation is a mystical experience in which we realize the paradoxical union of qualities such as "good" and "bad," or "love" and "hate," and ultimately the union of "ego" and "Self." To recognize the possibility of the resulting disorientation is to be prepared.

Transformation solves the problem posed by paradox, and is for this reason a wonderful experience. But when the dust settles the implications begin to impress themselves on us. Up to the point of transformation, our entire way of living has been based on the assumption that we are separate beings. The "ego" experiences itself as unique and individual, separate from the rest of the universe. This assumption usually structures and sustains our entire approach to life, in our work, our play and our relationships; and we therefore normally give little consideration to issues much greater than our own personal needs. At a very deep level, however, it is this very assumption of separateness which leads us to illness; and this assumption which is forever altered by the transformational experience.

The "Self" experiences itself as inextricably part of something much greater. The Self relates to the whole, the universe, God, or transcendent being and is, in the mystical experience, what affirms a connection to our divinity. Illness begins when we lose or forget our connection to the Self. In Indian traditional medicine, this state is known as Pragyaparadh, meaning the "mistake of the intellect," because it is the function of the conscious intellect to create distinctions; and it is the intellect which forgets our essential connection to the whole, and is the source of our human arrogance. The experience of transformation is therefore a kind of remembering; a remembering of our true condition, which we have forgotten.

After the euphoria of transformation we may begin to see that healing is going to involve making some major changes in the way we live out our lives. A change in our most fundamental assumptions will quite naturally precipitate a change in our attitudes and behaviour, which will in turn have a profound impact on our work and relationships. The implications for our lives are urgent and irreversible. Turning back would mean an inevitable return to the illness we want to heal, and worse, a conscious and deliberate one.

In fact, to return knowingly to denial and to illness is nearly an impossible undertaking—we could not really do it even if we wanted to. Before transformation our state of forgetting was unconscious and we were unaware of our responsibility for our lives and our health. After transformation, we can never be irresponsible again without choosing it as a conscious act. Our new awareness of this weighty responsibility can be so awesome that we become overwhelmed with fear. With that fear comes tension, and with the tension back comes pain, and with the pain comes dis-ease, and with dis-ease comes the illness which only a short time before had disappeared. This devastating set-back has been acknowledged in the mystical concept of the "dark night of the soul," a phrase borrowed from the writings of the Spanish Christian mystic, St. John of the Cross, and somewhat altered to suit our purposes.

THE DARK NIGHT OF THE SOUL

The euphoric experience of transformation may last for quite some time, but it can also be the prelude to the dark night of the soul, a state of profound depression or alienation which seems endless. The concept of the "dark night" is found in much mystical writing and describes the ultimate paradox, the final hurdle before the attainment of paradise. Often the experience is described in traditional literature as a "journey" over water at night in a frail boat, in which the traveller is totally at the mercy of the elements.

By relating these metaphors to illness and healing, we can bring the idea of the dark night into our immediate experience. At the point of transformation, we experience a state of union with a greater being, a taste of paradise so to speak, the elusive completion for which we are all striving in one way or another. Nonetheless, at just the moment paradise is attained, we go through the agony of realizing that we have lost it forever.

THE EXPLANATION

If the above description seems rather esoteric, we should realize that mystical experience engages the non-intellectual part of our being and it is only because we live so much in our heads that we require every experience to be tagged with some sort of rational explanation. Rationalization allows us to feel comfortable and "sane," and permits us to pass on our experience to others. Prior to transformation, we rationalize and encode our experience in ways which reflect both our childhood conditioning and the culture in which we are embedded. We recognize on some level that life is inexplicable, but act quite otherwise, as though pretending to ourselves that everything can be explained—despite all appearances to the contrary.

During the transformational experience, however, our intellect sustains a devastating assault. We suffer the dissolution of a lot of our old beliefs and flounder in a sea of paradox, often for a considerable time. As we view our experience in retrospect and the light of reason returns, several explanations and courses of action present themselves.

In his books on the teachings of Don Juan, Carlos Castenada describes being constantly put in unusual life situations, to which he could find no rational resolution. Apparently, Don Juan deliberately structured experiences which challenged Carlos's rational view of life, and then waited for his response to these situations to teach him new ways of relating to the world. In one passage, Don Juan refers to three bad habits which people get into to deal with such confrontations between the rational mind and life itself. He called them the bigot's way, the fool's way, and the pious man's way. Insinuating that Carlos himself appeared to favour the fool's way, Don Juan went on to suggest a more difficult fourth way, the warrior's way—or living life in the conscious acceptance of paradox. For Carlos, the problem of this fourth way was that it appeared to answer his questions by not answering them. With a little imagination we can redefine those categories in terms of the concepts we have considered in this book, and relate them to illness and to transformation.

1. DENIAL

After coming close to a transformational experience we can attempt to deny that it occurred, shore up the cracks in the old belief system, and return to our previous behaviour patterns. Don Juan would have called this the bigot's way. The reversal must of necessity be a "conscious" rejection of our experience, and so amounts to a further imposition of intellectual control over feeling.

Denial occurs when we are so fearful of the process of transformation that the ego sees no choice but to defend itself absolutely. This situation is a tragedy for all concerned. Such intellectual rejection of the transformational experience is often justified by blaming the institution or organization which "put us through" the experience.

Rather than acknowledge the fear in ourselves, we project our problem onto those attempting to facilitate our transformation, heaping our anger on them rather than ourselves. In this way the "ego" maintains a position of nonresponsibility, and can return to its previous perception of the world.

Allegations of charlatanism and malpractice come from this kind of patient, making them a source of concern and fear for those practitioners involved in new medicine. Unfortunately, there is no way out of this dilemma. To be effective in transformational therapy, we must work so close to people's denied negativity that we continually risk this kind of reaction. We must confront our own fear, however, if we are to help others confront theirs. Unfortunately, however, when people consciously refuse the transformational journey, they also lose the opportunity to heal, and everybody loses. It is a no-win situation. The price of rejection and continued denial is a return to illness, but with a difference. The ego is now better defended, and so less likely than ever to discover the healer within.

2. THE TREATMENT JUNKIE

Other people find that they have had a powerful experience, but are not able to leave it alone and move on. Such people seem to become stuck in a state of worry and obsession. Don Juan would have called this course the fool's way. There is no question of a rejection of the experience—in fact quite the opposite has occurred.

If we think the experience itself is the answer to our problems, and forget the lesson it could have taught us, we are enmeshed in the fool's trap. We think that because we are not fully healed we must keep looking for another similar experience, or even that we must keep repeating the same experience over and over. The focus is entirely on the memory of the experience itself, which of course is in the past, rather than staying in the present, which—

ironically—was exactly the lesson to be learned from the experience.

By becoming stuck in the early stages, we prevent ourselves from entering the dark night and lose the opportunity to heal. If our intellects are allowed to work over the experience obsessively, we risk getting stuck in the process, channeling the transformative energy which could take us forward into fueling an intellectual merry-go-round. People in that situation may go from therapist to therapist looking for the elusive experience which will finally "clear out their blocks," and become addicted to the experience in the same way that they may have been addicted to other behaviours or substances. They become treatment junkies. Unfortunately, their healing is necessarily deferred to another day.

3. THE CLOSED EXPLANATION

Our third option is to adopt a new set of beliefs to explain our experience. We can authorize someone, something, or some organization to explain the experience for us so that we feel to have "the" answer. Don Juan would have called this choice the pious man's explanation. Religions, science, or medicine itself can become the focus of such newborn beliefs. But in giving authority to an external explanation, we unwittingly deny our own authority and integrity. Such relinquishment of authority is only another kind of denial, and its price may be continued illness.

The attraction of a closed set of beliefs as explanation is its safety. If everything is explained in advance, we imagine we can largely avoid the sensation of being cast adrift on a dark and tempestuous sea. The danger, of course, is that we trade the possibility of spiritual growth, for present safety and limits.

Many people with chronic illness have been searching for answers for some time before they come to our clinic and have often been attracted to one or another of the plethora of theories which seek to explain the problems of our existence. Some clients therefore come into our program having adopted a new closed belief system. Unfortunately, whatever explanation they have found has left them still ill and looking for effective therapy.

These patients can be difficult to help because they cannot consider the possibility that their need for a closed explanation may be part of their problem. Any such suggestion is vigorously denied—a clue that we are pressing on a painful area. Like it or not, when we adopt someone else's explanation of reality we only discover another way of defending our ego, religious faith being, famously, a nearly impenetrable one.

4. THE OPEN EXPLANATION

The last option is an open explanation—the paradoxical notion that an explanation is not needed. We cannot get away from explanations altogether, because even no explanation is an explanation. But we can at least remain open to new ideas and perceptions whenever we come across them. Openness allows us to remain flexible, so that we do not develop the rigidity which initially led to our illness.

We must challenge ourselves to face our own despair—the despair of having nowhere to stand and no possibility of ever finding any solid ground—if we are to remain open and non-judgemental. Don Juan would have called this the warrior's way, or the way of accepting paradox for the mystery it is and moving forward. It is both the dark night of the soul, and the way to freedom and paradise. It is despair and elation, health and illness, everything contained in nothing—the essence of wholeness. By choosing the warrior's alertness, flexibility and body-mind balance, we may be able to fully comprehend the healing experience.

The idea that to remain healthy we must give up all need to explain the nature of our existence is the ultimate slap in the face to the intellect and the ego. Most of us have spent our lives building up inventories of information and "facts," only to discover that in the end we must throw it all away. Freedom is only gained after a long struggle with the need to know something concrete, and accepting the final realization that nothing is really known, and that nothing really needs to be known. The dark night of the soul only ends when we realize that it will never end. Paradise is not a place which we can get to through some formula or other, but it is a way of being here and now, of living without those artificial barriers which destroy our essential wholeness. To live in this way we must be greater than contradiction, and be able to contain the contradiction within the totality of who we are.

The totality is larger than our intellect, not the other way around, and so it is our ego which must give up its treasured position at the top of the heap. The universe contains mysteries which we will never understand. But one thing we can try to understand is that there *is* no objective reality out there which is in any way separate from us as observers. The observer and the observed are part of the same continuum. We are simply our-Selves, watching our-Selves, working with our-Selves, playing with our-Selves, creating our reality as we go forward together into the unknown. In a sense, there is nothing that is *not* a mystery. That is "reality" as we can know it. To live fully we must come to terms with an ultimate reality, where health merges with illness, the known merges with the unknown, and death merges with life.

Chapter Twenty

THE ENERGY BUCKET

Waste not, want not

*I*n this chapter, we want to suggest a simple blueprint which can help us stay healthy for the rest of our lives. Paradoxically, the task is both simple and impossible—simple because the art of staying healthy really is simplicity itself, impossible because in the end there can never be any blueprint or prescription to accomplish it.

So far this book has documented a series of insoluble but richly instructive paradoxes and has postulated that underlying chronic illness is a culturally induced mind-set. Unable as a society to accept and integrate the paradoxical nature of our existence, we seem to have forgotten as individuals our connection to a larger "Self"—and the interconnectedness of all life—and instead have emphasized our separateness. As a result, our idea of how life should be is at variance with the way it actually is. We are at odds with the truth of our existence, and cannot deal with the contradiction without challenging our intellect's supremacy.

We have also noted that our medical system has grown out of the same cultural mind-set which has put us individually at odds with ourselves, and so naturally reflects its limitations, becoming a major factor in the genesis of the very illnesses it tries to treat. And throughout the book, of course, we have discussed the need for a transformative journey and stressed the fact that since the intellect is unable to cope with paradoxes, such a journey must shift the locus of control from intellect to heart. Only the heart is capable of making decisions effortlessly, so that life can be lived in a more flexible way.

Without this fundamental shift of emphasis, our overburdened intellect must take increasing control of our decision-making, leading us to adopt a rule-centred approach to our lives which is ultimately destructive. As we have seen, we manifest this need to control, as a society, by making laws directed back at ourselves as individuals. These laws, however, are often experienced as conflicting with the requirements of a given situation; and over time, the effort to mold ourselves around such inappropriate and often inflexible rules becomes increasingly stressful.

In the last chapter, we touched briefly on yet another paradox, and one close to home. As authors, we face a writer's paradox. By writing—especially using traditional vocabulary and syntax, which themselves reflect our society's value system and logical bias—we are necessarily caught in a trap. We are condemned to try to intellectualize something which cannot at all be grasped by the intellect, and to try to describe it in language inherently hostile to its fundamental meaning. All in all, we can do little more than acknowledge that we are in fact helpless to "describe" any set of "rules" which will lead our readers to a healthy life.

THE QUANTUM BODY

Having said that it's impossible, however, let's nevertheless try to visualize, as simply as possible, the body as a dynamic process—a process which includes both structure and energy, intellect and feeling. Although the body appears to be a solid object, it is in fact principally a process—as we might define a fountain or a waterfall more by their dynamic processes, their action or continual movement, than by their constituent matter, water.

When we look at a fountain, we think we see an object. It has shape and structure which are dependent on the flow and pressure of the water passing through it. Similarly, our physical structure is dependent on the flow of energy and material passing through our bodies. There is a constant turnover of molecules and cells in our bodies so that over a period of time our material structure is completely refreshed. The cells of our stomach lining are replaced every three or four days; our livers are renewed every six weeks or so; even our bones, which seem so solid, are actually "fluid" in the sense that they are continuously renewed, completing a cycle every three or four years. In fact, in a scant seven years every atom in our bodies has been changed. Yet we retain our sense of personal identity as if nothing had happened.

The idea that the body is more flow than structure has been described in great detail by many authors. In *From Being to Becoming,* Nobel prize laureate Ilya Prigogine has developed a detailed theory of dynamic systems known as "dissipative structures." He sees these structures as non-living chemical systems which maintain themselves with an input and output of energy, thus exhibiting behaviours characteristic of life, such as metabolism, self-renewal, and evolution. Deepak Chopra, too, in his book *Quantum Healing* describes the "quantum mechanical body," in which thoughts, as the primary impulses, are the creative force which structure the body through the production of neuro-peptides.

But we don't really need a detailed scientific description of dissipative systems to appreciate the concept of energy flow. All we need do is picture ourselves as a flow of energy rather than as a static mass. With this simple understanding of the dynamics of our bodies, we possess all the information we need to maintain reasonable health.

Let's choose, then, the image of a bucket full of water to help illustrate structure and flow and their consequences for illness and health. The structural appearance of the body can be represented by the bucket and the dynamic aspect by the water contained in the bucket (*fig. 1*). In the bottom of the bucket is the karmic sediment representing our constitutional weaknesses, past indiscretions and genetic predispositions.

The debris piles up to form an uneven surface of bumps and hillocks on the bottom, but as these are usually covered by water, they lie unseen. The water level in the bucket represents the energy available to the individual at any given moment.

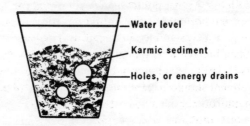

Fig. 1 The bucket full of water. The water level in the bucket represents our overall "energy state" at any given moment. Energy input must be equal to or greater than energy output if we wish to remain healthy

The basic concept of good health is to have our "energy bucket" full to overflowing at all times. Unfortunately, with the passage of time, the bucket gets kicked around and damaged by the abuses of the controlling intellect, and holes of varying sizes appear through which energy can escape. The holes can represent the wounds of the injured child, the stress of day-to-day living, and the unexpressed needs of the adult.

In short, anything denied or repressed represents a hole in the bucket, and drains energy from the system. During the first half of our lives, we usually have plenty of water in the bucket, and we are not concerned with our gradual loss of energy. However, as the water level drops lower, we begin to notice increasing fatigue. By this time our container has probably acquired multiple holes. We may begin then to wage a constant battle, pouring energy supplements—tonics, vitamins, drugs—into the bucket in order to keep the levels up, or continue to drain our resources by indulging in an unhealthy diet, heavy smoking, or too little sleep—in other words, generally neglecting ourselves.

Chronic fatigue now affects more and more people at earlier and earlier ages. If the water level gets too low, the sediment begins to show through, and we begin to have symptoms of illness. At that point we may panic and run to see the doctor, in the hope that she can find out what's causing the symptoms, and wave a magic wand to make our illness go away. Such behaviour implicitly misunderstands the nature of "cause." The tacit agreement between doctor and patient is that treatment should restore the smooth surface of the water, leaving the doctor no choice but to offer to remove any bumps, or symptoms, which happen to be visible above the surface. In other words, the doctor is expected to treat the symptoms; and if the treatment is superficially successful, we feel better, and go away without learning a thing, believing that all is well.

In this way we miss the essential message of our illness, which is that it is time to pay attention to the energy drains on our body-mind. Unfortunately, conventional medicine rarely addresses the problem of energy deficiency. Scientific medicine, because of its reductionist approach—its tendency to look at the body in pieces—really has no concept of an overall energy state, and therefore does not understand its impact on health.

Both doctor and patient understand the cause of illness to be the sediment which is showing through the surface of the water. In making this assumption, both participate in a delusion which is in essence part of a complex process of denial. They cling to this deception so that they can believe that the illness is "nobody's" "fault." It is so much easier to blame a microbe than to take responsibility for oneself and change one's habits. Denying the significance of our energetic situation, which is our responsibility, denies us both our power and our ability to effect change. Reason tells us that we cannot cause a viral infection—viruses do that; and a rear-end collision at a stop-sign—how could we be responsible for that. Reason, however, cannot see the whole truth.

It is low energy which permits infection and accidents. Let's continue our sketch of the overall holistic picture so that we will have something we can carry with us. Such an energetic analysis will not only empower us to be responsible for our own health, but offers a simple conceptual framework to explain how disease arises. Rather than focusing on the symptoms of illness, we can focus on increasing and maintaining the system's overall energy. There are obviously two ways of doing that. One is to increase the energy input, and the other is to reduce the energy output.

INCREASING ENERGY INPUT

First, a few words of caution regarding any method of improving one's health: any formula or therapy can become as stressful as the problem it is trying to correct if it is followed fanatically. Fanaticism of any type—whether it be for exercise, diet, energy balance or spiritual salvation—can in fact worsen a situation once the initial euphoria has worn off. It is no way to fill the energy bucket nor plug its leaks.

DIET

Though specific dietary programs are beyond the scope of this book, there are some general points about the modern food industry which are disturbing. For example, it has been suggested that recent changes in the structure of the gluten molecule may be causing increasing numbers of people trouble with the wheat products in their diets. It seems, too, that this altered gluten is also present in the meat of commercial livestock. If we couple this with the effects of residual pesticides, hormones, antibiotics, additives and microwave sterilization, we can see that our whole food chain has been altered by the agro-industry with little attention to the quality of the food itself. Even if the effects of such processing are only minimal, it would seem prudent to eat as organically as possible, and to limit our intake of processed foods.

But. An analysis of diet from an energetic standpoint might consider that, assuming our basic diet is at least reasonably sensible, worrying about what we should or shouldn't eat can actually drain more energy than an imperfect diet. So though the "pickup" often experienced when a new diet is first adopted can convince us that the whole answer to good health lies in diet, that conviction developed into an obsession can become harmful.

As diet-based health books are on every bookstand and the idea seems so reasonable, many people are caught in the trap of prescribing and dutifully pursuing various dietary restrictions and supplements for themselves. But a simple energetic analysis would suggest that there are considerations beyond proteins, fats, carbohydrates and vitamins. How we think about the food we eat and the act of eating, for instance, are vital. It is just as important to *enjoy* food as it is to eat the "correct" food.

Reverence for the food we eat can also make a life-giving difference to mere consumption. As Barry Holstun Lopez points out in his book, *Amaguk and Sacred Meat*, North-American Indians felt that buffalo meat was sacred if they had hunted and killed the buffalo themselves. They believed that there was a special relationship between hunter and hunted that endowed food with spiritual energy. It can be difficult for people who buy all their food off supermarket shelves to understand the difference between store-bought food and that which is personally produced—grown or hunted—but if there is something of the individual in the food he or she eats, that relationship will make available more of the food's beneficial energy when it is eaten. In other words, such food is "sacred."

Reverence for what we eat can be heightened in a number of other ways as well. Paying attention to our eating, rather than munching on a sandwich while driving to our next appointment; taking a moment to observe respect for food before beginning to eat; and taking the time to prepare our food ourselves, are all ways of increasing the vitality of our relationship to what we eat. Not incidentally, when we treat our food as sacred, and give it our full attention and respect, the tendency to eat in an unbalanced way is instinctively reduced, and the problem of "nutrition" in the sense of adequate fats, carbohydrates, and proteins, takes care of itself. The obsession with diets and eating evaporates, and that particular hole in the energy bucket is closed.

DIETARY SUPPLEMENTS AND TONICS

Many people these days resort to vitamins, tonics or food supplements when their bodies don't appear to be working properly. Supporting such habits is a rapidly expanding health food industry which thrives on fear of disease and desire for the health in a bottle. It would seem a real help if we could find a way to make the world of supplements a little less of a mystery.

Let's look to some simple energy principles to provide some straightforward answers. Traditional Chinese Medicine (TCM) maintains that whole plants have energies other than the caloric ones familiar to Western biochemists and weight-watchers. This other energy is known as "Qi."

The concept is the centuries-old basis of Traditional Chinese Medicine and is not dissimilar to the concept of "energy" as we are using it. The Chinese believed that extracting or isolating the various constituents of plants or herbs impaired or destroyed their Qi. This of course directly contradicts our practice of isolating and concentrating "active ingredients" from their sources. But conventional thinking has no concept comparable to "Qi," so cannot be used in energetic analyses.

The Chinese divided all plants or herbs into three categories:

Food grade plants which regenerate or build the body and which can be consumed regularly with no side-effects; *medicinal herbs* which can strengthen the body's functioning but which can have side-effects if eaten regularly; and *poisonous herbs* which must be used with extreme caution. The power of these can be further enhanced by mixing or combining different whole plants together to form specific energetic formulae.

This classification contains a couple of important concepts. First, food is seen as regenerative, while medicinal herbs are understood to be substitutes for or aids to the body's natural functions. Second, it is the "whole" herb or food which has the Qi and its strengthening properties, not any isolated extract which is called for. In other words, the difference between taking vitamin C in capsules and eating fruit which contains the vitamin is profound. An extract may well seem to have more concentrated therapeutic value, but the isolation of the active principles eliminates its original energy. Its Qi is gone.

Our conventional medical practice seems a double-edged sword—we enhance one property at the expense of another. This might explain why many supplements seem to lack the very strengthening we want from them—"energy"—and give us the one thing which we do not want, "side-effects," a consequence almost unknown when whole medicinal herbs are used judiciously. Moreover, our bodies can become weakened by, and possibly even dependent on, such extracts. Nevertheless, we have gone so far with the process that nowadays we even extract individual amino acids from protein molecules which themselves have been isolated from the whole food.

We are not suggesting that all extracts are harmful—far from it—but why spend a lot of money on expensive extracts when the original organic food is much cheaper and its safety is without question? Common sense alone indicates that some important questions need to be asked about taking food supplements. First, is the supplement whole natural food or an isolated element? Second, is the plant medicinal or food-grade? And third, has the natural food been enhanced with other whole foods or have its active principles been extracted and concentrated? If a supplement is made from whole, food-grade herbs, the natural energy is probably intact and will likely be beneficial to our energy state. At worst, being food, it can't do us much harm.

Furthermore, while there may be nothing wrong with a particular supplement, particularly if it is a whole food, our energy bucket sketch can show us how very limited taking supplements alone to correct health problems really is. First, filling up the bucket with more water can only be a tempo-rary measure if there are a lot of holes in the bucket. The energy level can be kept a little higher, granted, but as long as there are substantial holes in the bucket, we must keep pour-ing more and more in to keep the level up; and what started as a little vitamin supplement can eventually turn us into a walking pharmacopoeia. Second, spending money and en-ergy and pinning our hopes on tonics and supplements re-sults in a new energy drain—particularly if the supplement is an isolate with little energetic value. In short, dosing our-selves in this way can make existing holes bigger, so that more supplements are needed. The net result is that tonics alone cannot work.

SUPPLEMENTS AND SUBJECTIVE FEEDBACK

Many people habitually swallow tonics, vitamins and die-tary supplements of all kinds without having any way of knowing whether they are improving their health or not. We therefore urgently need some way to assess the value of what we are putting into our bodies. Without such a gauge we must rely on our doctor, nutritionist or herbalist to "prescribe" the right therapy without our informed feedback. Not to mention that this blind reliance on outside authority is, as we've seen, itself just another hole in the bucket.

So unless we are very careful and proceed with a great deal of self-awareness the practice of supplementation can be fraught with negative energetic consequences. Time out for relaxation and introspection, aided by some form of meditation (see further below) can make a crucial difference to self-awareness and so to our understanding of our health and the effects, good or bad, of treatments. The paradox here is that if we *had* this sort of self-awareness we would probably not be ill.

EXERCISE

Everybody knows that regular exercise is a good thing, and doctors often recommend exercise programs they feel are appropriate to their patients' continued health or comeback from illness. We are all familiar with the heart patient who, after his recovery, is seen regularly walking the neighbourhood streets, performing his daily one- or two-mile constitutional.

Exercise is a wonderful thing; it tones the body inside and out and keeps it fit. As we all know, too, the body over time will actually change shape to accommodate an exercise regularly performed—the very image of the quantum or fluid body. And although exercise uses energy, it also works to release or create more than it consumes. This energy creation seems a paradox in itself. How can something that uses energy produce energy? There is no easy answer to the question, except to say that the experience is common and universal. Certainly as the body becomes fitter it becomes more efficient in using energy. And perhaps exercise in clearing the mind simply makes us feel more alive.

As with diet, however, our state of mind while exercising, though often overlooked, is very important. If we really don't feel like exercising, or if we exercise too much, exercise like anything else can become an energy drain.

It is important therefore to choose exercise we really enjoy. After all, if we don't enjoy what we are doing we are unlikely to persist with it. Yet how many people consider this point? How many joggers do we see struggling through their last mile with a look of desperation on their faces, hating every minute of it, yet doing it because they feel they should, or because they must beat yesterday's time?

When the intellect says we must exercise, but feeling says "I don't like it," a conflict arises in the body which is stressful and energy draining. Exercise performed under those circumstances can actually be harmful. When the intellect and the feeling are at odds, there is a hole in the bucket, and energy drains out. When the mind and body are in agreement the holes are closed.

REST

Rest is the body's "down-time," a time in which to sit back, sleep, do nothing or take stock of events. In a culture which pressures us to do as much as possible, and penalizes us for resting, many of us get so busy with our various commitments that we never get adequate rest. Interns, for example, often work as much as thirty-six hours at a stretch without sleep, ironically proposing to learn to heal others while ignoring their own body's needs.

That the medical establishment should perpetuate a practice so grossly destructive to the health of new doctors is quite bizarre. But as it is taboo to question tradition and the wisdom of superiors, most interns push the problem aside and carry on, in an effort to "prove" themselves. After all, the profession is really only a reflection of our entire culture, riddled as it is with competitiveness and the work ethic and the imbalances they generate. And as a society, we are profoundly rest-deprived.

Healthy living means being aware of our own needs while we move and interact with others in the world. Though many of us have been taught that looking after our own needs before others' is wrong, and suffer intolerable guilt at the mere thought of such "selfish" behaviour, the problem with neglecting ourselves while looking out for others is that it doesn't work.

Self-inflicted pressure is generally one of the biggest holes in our bucket and rapidly leads to illness. Paradoxically, illness so acquired relieves us of the guilt we would feel for looking after ourselves in the first place. So a breakdown produces enormous benefit by solving an insoluble problem—how else can we look after ourselves without feeling guilty? Given such a benefit from illness, it is hard to see why anyone would want to get well. To correct this problem we have to realize that it is not selfish to be self-aware. The paradox of healthy living and giving is that we can only give of ourselves if our own bucket is full to overflowing. We must give from a state of fullness rather than of depletion, or suffer the inevitable consequences.

MEDITATION

One way to resolve the problem of inadequate rest is to structure regular rest periods into the day. A variety of techniques which train the mind and body to slow down all answer to the name of "meditation." Ideally, the mind ceases its incessant chatter and becomes quiet, allowing deep rest on all levels of our being.

The meditative state is one of restful alertness. We are conscious and awake, but not necessarily thinking of anything in particular. We are awake to ourselves only, turned inwards. EEG studies performed on meditating subjects show increased alpha-wave activity in the brain, and increased coherence of electrical activity in its two hemispheres.

In his book, *The Maharishi Technology of the Unified Field: The Neurophysiology of Enlightenment,* Dr. Robert Wallace outlines much of the research done in the last twenty years on transcendental meditation. Meditation rests the body even more profoundly than sleep. Metabolic rates, for example, fall lower than during sleep, and breathing is lessened. Numerous studies have demonstrated meditation's beneficial effects on stress-related disorders such as asthma, hypertension, anxiety, hypercholesterolaemia and depression. It's hard to believe that a practice so universally beneficial is not a standard therapeutic tool, while tranquilizers and antidepressants are widely and casually used. But in spite of the evidence, the medical profession does not normally endorse meditation. Nor does it conceive of providing time for hospital staff to meditate.

Meditation is a powerful tool both for filling the bucket, and for sealing its leaks. Periods of structured introspection allow us to become aware of the energetic configuration of our bodies, and to use our minds to affect that configuration. During meditation, insights into deep-seated childhood pain may arise spontaneously and feelings buried or walled-off for fear of their inappropriateness may surface, and so be released. This freeing of energy seals holes in our energy bucket with the result that there is a gradual movement towards greater wholeness of mind, body and spirit, and over time, increasing awareness is accompanied by measurable rejuvenation from deep rest.

Unfortunately, few people will take up meditation before they have had a transformational experience, as silent contemplation is judged to be both self-centred and useless, and guilt prevents us from taking time for our own needs. Sitting doing "nothing" for hours can hardly solve the problems of the world, it might seem! But in fact the altered perception acquired through transformation clearly links the problems of the world to too much activity engendered by a society motivated by guilt and fear. To sit in meditative silence, then, rejuvenating ourselves and renewing our energy might actually be the ultimate act of healing both for us as individuals and for our planet.

CLOSING THE HOLES

We cannot regain our health completely without making some attempt to close the holes in our bucket. In fact, if closing the holes were all that we did—even if we never attempted to refill the bucket—we would in time recover simply because the very acts of eating, breathing and sleeping put more energy into our system. But closing the holes can seem a daunting task. Ultimately, we will be required to abandon our defences, and our denial, to face the fear of our helplessness, and risk the annihilation of the transformational moment before embarking on a healing journey. However, if we are prepared to do this, the reward is that closing the holes can become almost effortless and even enjoyable. Whenever we let go, problems bubble up without difficulty, and in so doing they almost solve themselves.

To look for healing through inner change rather than treatment is, as we have seen, already a step on the path to personal transformation. There are many opportunities in this day and age to pursue the self-understanding necessary to begin the process. That is, the motivation to begin healing does not have to be critical illness, though most of us seem to need to be confronted by a serious problem before we will face the challenge of transformation. Illness usually poses that kind of problem, though ultimately every interactive experience can be used as an opportunity to close holes.

Relationship is an interaction between two energy fields leading to a certain outcome, positive or negative—whenever we interact with another we come away feeling better or worse. If a relationship constantly produces anxiety or difficulty, it is a hole in the bucket through which energy leaks out. With this understanding, difficult relationships can be transformed into opportunities for healing rather than static situations of continuing warfare. Instead of running away, we can use difficulties for the gift which they really are—guides to the hitherto hidden holes in our bucket. How many marriages would be saved if people understood that simple point!

Eventually, the realization that consciousness is at the root of all our experience will itself fuel our desire to continue to expand our consciousness and continue our transformational experience. And gradually we will discover that ultimately, *every* experience is an opportunity to heal.

Chapter Twenty-one

WHOLENESS, PHYSICIANS AND PATIENTS

The whole is in the part; the part contains the whole

*T*he book of Genesis, which describes the Christian version of the creation myth, opens with a very familiar story. The story of the Garden of Eden focuses on the miraculous tree, known as "the Tree of the Knowledge of Good and Evil" which grew at its very centre, and on God's stern prescription against Adam and Eve's eating its fruit, on pain of death; and of course on the Serpent, whose skills in elementary logic seem to have changed the course of human destiny.

There are many different versions of the myth and some are more elaborate than others. In one version, the Serpent pushes a cautious but curious Eve against the Tree and taunts her, saying, "Look! touching the Tree won't hurt you, so how can the fruit do you any harm?" Poor Eve, however, comprehends immediately the harm such questioning of authority has brought them all when she recognizes the figure of Death coming toward them. Frightened, and understanding her mortality, she realizes that as the "mother of all living," she must now also "enlighten" Adam and all of creation. So it is said that Eve then picked fruit from the tree and ate it, asking Adam and all the animals and birds of the Garden to do the same. And it is said that all but the phoenix tasted the fruit, and that is why it alone still enjoys immortality.

Genesis also tells us that after Adam and Eve had eaten the fruit of the Tree of the Knowledge of Good and Evil, they noticed they were naked, and were ashamed and covered themselves with fig leaves; and when at dusk God walked in the Garden, he found them hiding from his gaze. And God confronted them, asking, "Who told you of your nakedness? You must have eaten of the forbidden tree," whereon Adam tried to exonerate himself, saying, "Don't blame me, Eve made me do it" and Eve, sighing heavily, also attempted to excuse herself, saying, "Don't blame me, it was the Serpent that beguiled me." But God was not to be appeased. He was so upset that he cursed the three of them with dreadful consequences for their disobedience. To the Serpent he said, "You shall lose your legs, and writhe on your belly forever, eating dust. And there shall be a lasting enmity between you and the woman's children. They will stamp on the heads of your children until their heels are bruised." Then he cursed Eve, saying, "I will greatly increase your pain in childbearing, yet you shall yearn for your husband, and be ruled by him." Next he turned to Adam saying, "Because you have obeyed her rather than me, the ground is cursed because of you, and you shall eat bread in the sweat of your brow, struggling to uproot thorns and thistles from it. Dust you are, and dust you'll return to when you die."

Now in the Garden was another tree known as the Tree of Life. This Tree was reputed to confer immortality on anyone who ate its fruit. To prevent Adam and Eve from eating its fruit, God then drove them from the Garden forever, posting a whirling flaming sword in the east to bar the way in.

On the face of it, the Bible's first story seems to recount an angry God's punishment of his subjects for their transgression of his authority. But suppose we look at it from a different perspective, defining the various characters as parts of our individual consciousness, just as we have done with other tales elsewhere in this book. In such a reading, we might take the Garden of Eden to represent wholeness, a physical embodiment of the notion that everything in the universe is part of one great whole. Adam whose susceptibility to logical argument proves his downfall, might represent the intellect; Eve, who simply obeys the intellect's suggestion, our physical or emotional nature; and the Serpent, a curious and complex character in the story, might be said to represent the negative aspect of our intellect: that pride in our mind's abilities which beguiles us into thinking that we can know "everything." Significantly, this was exactly the claim of Francis Bacon, the father of our modern science.

Eating the fruit of the Tree of the Knowledge of Good and Evil might be said to give us the instinct and the ability to differentiate good from bad, and presumably illness from health. With a little imagination, then, we can read an understanding of the "genesis" of illness into the story of Adam and Eve. The most significant factor in the story seems to be the terrible consequences of acquiring the ability to discriminate. Seeing differences, and judging them "good" or "evil," seems the inevitable prelude to the loss of wholeness, putting us beyond the pale of Paradise on earth. But let's stop a moment to consider the opposite inference, which is quite remarkable: if we learn to transcend our innate ability to discriminate and find some way to stop seeing only the differences between things, it may be possible to regain our wholeness.

There are some other fascinating points in the story. Eve's punishment for learning to discriminate is, most notably, that she will be ruled by her husband—and, as she is now conscious of such differences, will understand her subjection for what it is. At the same time, it seems she is condemned to pine for the partner now so irrevocably separated from her, and for the equality which formerly defined their marriage. Not surprisingly, she will suffer to bear the offspring of such an unequal union. These punishments affect them both. Far from justifying a patriarchal society, we might understand such a curse to mean that in an imperfect or "fallen" world, hierarchical structures oppress us all, entrenching an unworkable and destructive imbalance, or dis-ease, in the very fabric of our daily lives.

Adam's fate is necessarily parallel. God sentences him to struggle and sweat every day of his life just to keep himself alive—the inference being that unceasing struggle is the automatic and inescapable result of the perception of differences. The work ethic in our society mimics this curse exactly, crushing the emotional natures of men and women, condemning many people to struggle all their lives without ever managing to feel worthy or adequate to their task. Interestingly, Adam is additionally cursed in that his death is absolute, dust to dust, whereas the woman's seems mitigated by her ability to bear children.

Another unmistakeable feature of the story is the eagerness of each of the "sinners" to blame someone else for their transgression. The buck stops at the Serpent—the original scapegoat. It seems God never thinks to ask what possessed one of his creatures to precipitate the genesis of sin, of disobedience to our higher good. He condemns such intellectual pride—that pride that makes us imagine ourselves as all-knowing as a god—cursing the Serpent to go on its belly in the dust for all time. The lasting enmity his curse foresees between such negative impulses and humankind itself can be witnessed in our tendency to blame one—*external*—"evil" or another for our ills. We do not seem to recognize that this "evil" was there in the beginning, an original and significant inhabitant of Eden, part of our primal wholeness, not an outside force at all. Finally, the phoenix, which would not eat the fruit, seems to represent our potential for transformation and healing, that potential which lies like a sleeping beauty in all of us.

The story of Adam and Eve, then, can be read as a challenge to return to Eden, to reintegrate ourselves in our original state of wholeness. Before embarking however, we should realize that the myth also states that the return to Eden will not be easy. God has forbidden us the Garden for our sin of intellectuality and pride, and the route back in seems certain death by a whirling flaming sword—

guaranteed to strike fear into the bravest. On reflection, however, we might realize that we have met such death-like barriers before, in fact repeatedly so, in other chapters in this book. Such barriers to the return to wholeness we have discovered represent the passage through a phase transition, an experience which *seems* like certain death at the outset, but which represents nothing more or less than a radical transformation and new life, comparable to the phoenix's death and rebirth in flames.

HOLISM

Holistic theory holds that human beings exist as individual points of awareness within a conscious universe, and as such we are already "whole." In "Auguries of Innocence," William Blake wrote,

> To see a World in a grain of sand
> And Heaven in a wild flower
> To hold Infinity in the palm of your hand
> And Eternity in an hour

A "world in a grain of sand" and "Infinity in the palm of your hand" are the very image of the holistic perception—each part of the whole also contains, and is, itself, the whole. Anything in the universe is therefore at once: a whole entity within that universe; the universe itself; and a part of that universe—just as the grain of sand is itself complete as a grain of sand, at the same time that it contains "a world" and is part of that world.

It would be difficult to conceive of a mightier paradox than this! Everything is whole in itself and at the same time part of an infinite number of other wholenesses. Such a view is really no different from the systems theory we mentioned earlier, however, which sees individuals as systems made up of smaller systems, which are at the same time part of larger systems. Still, such concepts confound our rational minds which are conditioned to deny one or the other of two contradictory principles.

Holism is essentially an extremely simple idea, albeit with awesome implications. For instance, if everything is already whole, then it follows that nothing need be done in order to achieve wholeness. At first glance, such a proposition seems reasonable. But then what about illness? It is natural to assume that if we are ill we must be less than whole. Both doctors and patients alike make that assumption. But if wholeness is an intrinsic attribute of everything in the universe, we *must still be whole even when we are sick!*—which seems to imply that we need no healing.

How is it possible to reconcile the paradox that we are both "whole" and "not whole" at the same time? The great gift of paradox is—whether in the form of a Zen koan, or Christian theology's three-gods-in-one—is that our very grappling with it ultimately forces us to the realization that either/or propositions cannot represent reality. Logical reasoning is its own limitation. Paradox and contradiction exist in the universe, and rationality must eventually bow to the fact.

The discoveries of the new physics which we discussed earlier also assert that both aspects of a paradox can and do co-exist; and point out that we see the one we set the experiment up to see—the one we want to see. Illness itself, then, is only a perspective, an attitude born of the denial of our intrinsic wholeness, which wants to see a part of itself as "bad" or to be rejected. Just as in a scientific experiment, if we take the point of view that we are not whole, then we are by definition "ill," but if we take the point of view that we are whole, then we are well.

DENIAL

Wholeness is our primal situation, our individual Garden of Eden. Denial is the conscious or unconscious mechanism which negates that wholeness. It is the splitting off of a part of the self and the refusal to acknowledge its existence. The "fall" from wholeness is our denial of a part of ourselves, that reflection of our distorted perception of ourselves which in turn manifests itself in a physical illness, representing—or "standing in for"— what has been denied.

The notion of wholeness seems very difficult to understand and assimilate intellectually. Paradoxically, it is its very simplicity that boggles the minds of most doctors and patients leaving us floundering in a sea of contradictions. But rather than getting tied up in logical knots, let's look at our personal experience of disease *(fig. 1)*.

WHOLENESS   DENIAL   ILLNESS

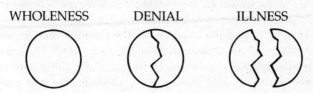

Figure 1—The development of illness through the process of denial.

When illness arises through denial, the desire to eradicate it is really an attempt to permanently "kill" the denied portion of the self. To try to heal in that way is to engage in a power struggle with oneself, and that struggle against the self is ultimately the nature of illness. In other words, the *struggle* to get better is in fact the very problem which created the illness in another guise. Struggle causes illness, it does not cure it.

Healing is therefore something entirely different from what we are conditioned to imagine. Amazing as it may seem, the assumption of their patients' *wholeness*, or "rightness," not a lack of them, is taken for granted by all successful healers as fundamental to the healing relationship. Healing in this context becomes not the removal of symptoms, but the re-integration of a rejected part of ourselves. Between healer and healed, then, illness has no absolute existence. It can in fact be said to be an "illusion"—not in the sense that it does not exist at all, but in that it only exists relative to health.

RECONSTITUTING WHOLE CONSCIOUSNESS

We can tell our attitude as individuals simply by examining exactly how we feel when we "fall" ill. Most people's natural reaction is, "I don't want this, please make it go away." But if illness is perpetuated by an inner power struggle, another paradox takes hold. Cause becomes effect and effect becomes cause.

Understanding this challenge to the long-held assumption that illnesses have discrete causes is absolutely crucial. When the self is at war with the self, the struggle is illness. The power struggle is there prior to the manifestation of symptoms, and *will still be there* even if the manifestation is somehow masked or removed. It is obvious, then, that any long-term solution to illness must deal with this struggle.

In the Judeo-Christian tradition, the notion of wholeness is represented by Eden and by heaven, and the loss of that wholeness by the Fall and by hell. But the ideas of wholeness, alienation and evil have been alluded to in virtually every spiritual tradition we know. Holism can seem superficially at odds with the dualistic notion of a spiritual war between good and evil, but in fact it does not deny this struggle. It simply points out that those who engage in the struggle against evil are actually expressing an overall cultural distortion and disregarding the biblical injunctions to "love thine enemy" and "resist not evil."

Reconstituting our wholeness is the spiritual quest or inner journey, then, to locate our denied or repressed parts and re-integrate them. Conventional medicine unfortunately no longer has any concept of wholeness. In fact, the mention of holism can upset physicians, who may see it as a threat to their turf. Though such a situation seems strange, it is just the way things are for the present, and reflects the imbalance in our overall world view.

Holistic medicine seeks to redress this imbalance. If physicians treat patients superficially, without dealing with the mind and the spirit, then they are in effect helping them to maintain their denial, and participating in their illness. No real healing can occur if physicians collude with patients in their struggle. Whatever good a particular treatment might do, illness will eventually arise again because the underlying distortion has not been addressed.

PHYSICIANS AND A THERAPEUTIC STRATEGY

To nudge patients toward healing, then, physicians must bring them to a confrontation with their denied self, then allow the energy of the denied part to do the talking and the healing. The physician's task is to recognize the wholeness already present, and assist the patient in recognizing it. Skilful physicians actually do very little else, understanding that interference only blocks the process of healing.

This does not mean that physicians should never act, but that they should feel less need to act in any given situation. Often patients will have their own solutions if their physician understands that illness has a message, and allows it to speak for itself. To do that, however, physicians must first understand that the illness is part of the patient's gestalt.

Truly assisting the healing process is not so much a matter of "acting," but of "not acting," or "being." Certain techniques, such as acupuncture, can catalyze the confrontation with denial, but they are not crucial. The only crucial thing is that the physician understand and incorporate holistic thinking into his or her very being, and act from a state of wholeness during the office interview.

Obviously, acquiring the healing attitude requires self-understanding, or as the saying goes, "physician heal thyself." To act from wholeness, physicians must have made the same attitudinal shift they will assist their patients in achieving (fig. 2). Not incidentally, physicians who become aware of their own wholeness, benefit enormously in their own lives—suffering far less stress and getting much more enjoyment from their work, finding that many of the problems which normally stress the busy physician simply disappear.

· CONVENTIONAL ASSUMPTIONS	· ASSUMPTIONS OF HEALING
· need to do something	· no need to act
· need to be knowledgeable	· no need to pretend to know everything
· need to make a diagnosis	· no need to look for diagnoses which are not there
· need to take responsibility	· no assumption of physician responsibility

Figure 2—showing the alternate view that physicians can take to facilitate the healing process.

HOLISM AND THE OFFICE INTERVIEW

The assumption that patients are intrinsically whole suggests a number of possible office interview techniques which to conventional thinking might seem absurd. The general thrust of the holistic interview is to generate a meeting between patient and illness. Since the illness is part of the personality of the patient, it can be treated as if it was itself a personality. Questions like: "What do you think the problem is trying to say to you" will often open the door to a discussion of the meaning of the illness in the context of the patient's life and relationships.

Many patients, however, will reply, "I've no idea— you're the doctor, you tell me." Though such deference to authority is part of the conditioning of our society—as Genesis makes perfectly clear—physicians must beware of patients who have discovered that it also serves them perfectly as a vehicle for transferring responsibility. Such a reply, veiled in the guise of deference, in fact allows patients to give absolute responsibility to their physicians, and deny their own accountability for their illness.

Such patients have often spent a lifetime developing techniques of denial and are likely to be masters at the

game. Illness always belongs to the patient, however, and
doctors must learn to give it back to them, or watch the
physician-patient relationship turn into a kind of tennis
game, in which the illness is passed fruitlessly back and
forth. Assuming the physician is aware there is a game of
tactics going on, an effective reply to such an initial volley
might be, "You are the person with the problem, not me.
If the illness were trying to give you a message, what do
you think it might be?"

Though standard practice dictates that physicians take
on patients for life, promising to look after every ailment
as it arises, this practice in fact actively disempowers their
patients rather than helping them, by suggesting that
healing comes from some external source. With time and
experience, astute healers will find any number of ways to
give illness back to their patients. As they work, their intuition will begin to generate appropriate questions or
thoughts in the context of particular healing relationships.
For example, as it is usually our emotional nature which is
suppressed, questions which connect "feeling" and
"illness" tend to put patients in touch with their denied
selves. The "right" comment delivered at the "right" moment, with the "right" amount of empathy, will open the
deep well of repressed feeling which, when released,
leads to the healing experience.

The art of the healer, then, lies not in diagnosis and
treatment, but principally in developing empathetic intuition. And to do that, physicians must learn to trust their
own feelings—such as anger and sadness—in the context
of the doctor-patient relationship, and allow them expression. They must stop pretending to be objective scientists
and understand that they are human beings in a critical
relationship.

No healing can ever occur if the healer is not coming
from her own truth. Physicians must take down the barriers, take off the white coats and participate in the healing
relationship as living beings. To do this, they must act
from their own woundedness; and when they do, the effect

is on their patients is instantaneous. Perhaps so many physicians feel threatened by holistic medicine because this shift away from their omnipotence also means questioning the very foundation of much of their training in objective scientific medicine and their own spiritual and emotional health.

DOROTHY

Dorothy was a woman with intractable "tennis elbow," who came to see us after she developed a painful flexion contracture which left her unable to straighten her arm. The problem had persisted despite all the conventional treatments for the condition and she wanted to try acupuncture. During the initial interview, she volunteered that her mother had been diagnosed with Alzheimer's disease at about the same time she developed the trouble with her elbow. Physically there was no conceivable connection between the two incidents, yet the interviewer's intuition prompted him to ask, "Do you think there is any connection between the elbow problem and your mother's Alzheimer's?" At this, Dorothy suddenly burst into tears and all her trepidation over her mother's diagnosis came pouring out. It turned out that she was desperately afraid of getting ill and in particular of developing Alzheimer's as her mother had done. When the fear was uncovered and released, recovery was rapid. Acupuncture was incidental.

Few text-books suggest that probing the meaning of diseases in close relatives is an effective treatment for tennis elbow, and rightly so. It is not a treatment, but an essential adjunct to diagnosis and discovery, without which no treatment regimen can ever be truly effective. The insight Dorothy had into the connection between her mind and body brought about rapid recovery of her tennis elbow. Without that insight, all physical therapies were likely to fail, as they had in the past.

THE ROLE OF FEAR

Dorothy's problem was obviously a deep-seated fear—a fear she then projected onto something outside of herself. Fear is often the energetic imbalance underlying denial; and our inability or unwillingness to fully experience it prevents a natural and spontaneous return to wholeness. In other words, it is our terror of being consumed by the whirling sword of flame which prevents our return to Eden.

Fear is the barrier, then, which prevents wholeness. If it is denied, it is either projected outside the self onto something else, or hidden in disease; and that disease or fear can then function as a rational *explanation* for and displacement of the "primal anxiety" Rollo May has noted we all feel. In other words, illness can become a focus for the projection of fear, and can absorb much of our existential anxiety. It is amazing how often a patient's anxiety disappears the moment an illness is diagnosed. In fact, many serious and even life-threatening physical illnesses—such as multiple sclerosis, systemic lupus erythematosus and cancer—are accompanied by a strange euphoria, as is much chronic pain. Small wonder then, that both illness and its cause must be rejected and located outside the self. Taking the illness back into the self requires accepting the anxiety again, after we have gone to so much trouble to get rid of it.

FEAR AND THE PHYSICIAN

While physicians may be quite able to see the fear mechanism operating in their patients, it's another matter altogether for them to turn inward and see the same mechanism operating in themselves. It seems a little known fact, but doctors are actually no different from anybody else! They share the same cultural tendencies and basic assumptions as the rest of society and therefore practise medicine with very much the same fear they encounter in their patients.

Defensive medicine—unnecessary or useless tests and procedures to avoid accusations of negligence—is just one of the results of this sort of fear. Physicians typically follow the rules as far as possible, justifying their conformity as essential to "maintaining good standards," when they are in fact acting defensively in order to avoid trouble. Fear, in other words, motivates much medical practice and prevents doctors from taking a common sense approach to people's problems. Much of what physicians do, therefore, may be no more than what they think they ought to. Patients by visiting their doctor are at least acknowledging that they have a problem, even if they are not willing to acknowledge the real problem.

When doctors then confine their attention strictly to physical symptoms, so as to avoid confronting their own or their patient's underlying fear, patients end up feeling unheard, frustrated, and ultimately, hostile. The consequence of that avoidance is likely to be an amplification of the original energetic imbalance. At the very least, the root problem the illness represents will be hurriedly masked rather than investigated.

Little wonder then that there is so little appreciation of the role of fear in disease. If patients project their fear onto their physicians, and physicians project their fear onto their patients, the result is a merry-go-round neither party can afford to acknowledge. The fear of lawsuits forces physicians to practise defensive medicine, and the practice of defensive medicine leads to suspicious patients who then are more likely to sue at the least provocation.

THE SOLUTION

As we are all sitting outside Eden, wanting to return to the state of wholeness it represents but unable to do so, what are we to do? One way out is to acknowledge our denial—we cannot expect to be whole if we persist in disowning parts of ourselves. And we might look to our physicians to do the same: to heal themselves before they offer to help anybody else. After all, no one can expect to pass on what they have not fully understood themselves.

The open acknowledgement of fear as a factor in disease would have profound implications for the doctor-patient relationship. For physicians, it would mean practising less defensive medicine, allowing themselves to be more human, and surrendering to their intuition. For patients it would mean admitting their personal responsibility for their illness and their health, and realizing that doctors don't have all the answers.

WHOLENESS, LIFE AND DEATH

Why did Eve notice Death approaching when she touched the Tree of Knowledge? The simple answer is that at the same moment we acquire the ability to discriminate, we must also confront the inevitability of death, life's necessary opposite. The unchangeable fact of existence is that we are born to die. Returning to wholeness therefore means regarding birth and death as equivalent.

Since it takes us back to the place where we began, death is really nothing to be afraid of. It is not something to be avoided or denied, but something to be accepted and, perhaps, like birth, even celebrated. Once we understand that, we can also see that true healing does not mean grasping at immortality, but rather, as physicians and patients alike so often forget, involves an acceptance of the limitations of our existence.

Tragically, our great common fear of dying not only creates much illness among us, but keeps us from living fully all aspects of our lives. The flaming sword whirls right in front of our eyes, daring our return to Eden, but we refuse even to look at it. All the while, the wholeness inherent in the Garden knows nothing of fear of death since it contains both and sees no difference between them.

The ultimate paradox is that to live fully, we must live in full awareness of our death from moment to moment. To achieve wholeness, we must centre our being in a place beyond the contradiction of life and death, illness and health, while embracing both. We must centre ourselves beyond all contradictions in fact, since they are all part of the overall wholeness. Wholeness is both the relative and the absolute; it is the root and the branch, the source of everything that exists, the beginning and the end of paradox.

ACKNOWLEDGEMENTS

We would like to thank the following people for their help and encouragement during the production of this book. First and foremost thanks go to our partners in life, Cherie Greenwood, who inspired us and suggested the title of this book and Heather Nunn, who gave us much encouragement and love to persist with it; Ruth Nadeau, whose meticulous reading inspired us to re-examine some of our erroneous notions regarding the English language; Tony Gregson, whose faith and perseverence allowed us to get the book into print; Miles Lowry, whose pictures seem to capture the magic of transformation; Jock Mckeen, Larry Dossey, Lieh Siebold, Don and June Mainwaring, June Cable, Sally Lang, Donna Dryer, Richard Jensen, and Linda Wyness for their help and constructive criticisms during the preparation of the manuscript; Michael Gregson and Susan Clark who took hold of the project at the later stages and pushed it to completion; our friends and supporters, Phyllis Kjellander, Bill Vogel, Sylvia Dixon, Miriam Myllymaki, Cathy Parr, and Karen Drysdale who helped us see the possible in the impossible; Joe Turner, Donna Ray, Bonita Mosdell, and Maureen McDowell, for their help with contracts and documents; Margaret Hincks and Mary Joan Zakovy for helping with corrections; Valerie Ryan, Ely and Joan Lawrence, Eileen Dunhé, and Claire Peterson, Bill and Catia Ryan, for their valuable help and advice with promotion and marketing.

Thanks go to all our teachers and patients who inspired most of the ideas which we have attempted to present; lastly to the universal spirit which provided words for our addled intellects to write down.

X

Y